# LAB TEST
## REFERENCES

**URVASHI PARMAR**

# RIGI PUBLICATION



## LAB TEST REFERENCES

By

URVASHI PARMAR



Originally published in India

ISBN: 978-93-88393-12-6 (Paperback)
978-93-88393-13-3 (eBook)

Published by RIGI PUBLICATION

777, Street no.9, Krishna Nagar

Khanna-141401 (Punjab), India

Website: www.rigipublication.com

Email: info@rigipublication.com

Phone: +91-9357710014, +91-9465468291

# Preface

In this book I have depicted many functions like Biochemistry, Microbiology, Hematology, Serology and Histology. Many of discrepancies are in medical field, yet Laboratory reports are final to judge to resolve that discrepancy, here I am trying to clear many topics via some reference reports and theory. Every topic has been designed to equipped young students with much knowledge on all topics as is desirable from the point of view of brilliant success in laboratory test.

Laboratory reports are more essential and important in medical sector. Its values and function must be clear and proper. Given values and composition are based on experiences and basic medical data.

# Dedication

I have great pleasure to dedicate this reference book to all Laboratory Technicians as well as Students.

# INDEX

# LABORATORY MANAGEMENT

## 1. Sample login

- Patient registration
- Sample identification
- Patient barcode
- Sample acceptance
- Sample rejection

## 2. Work assignment:-

- Sample organized
- Work list
- Work load list
- Sample scheduling

## 3. Result entry:-

- Manual & automatic calculation

## 4. Review & approval:-

- Repeat tests
- First review
- Result validation

## 5. Reports & Queries:-

- Trend analysis
- Test statistics
- Turnaround time

# INTRODUCTION TO MEDICAL LABORATORY

- MLT or DMLT is a basic course that equips the student with the most essential knowledge and skill certain to medical laboratories such as;-

- Importance of laboratory service
- Role of medical laboratory technologist
- Prevention and control of laboratory accidents
- Play a major role in patient care

**Laboratory organizational department:-**

- Clinical biochemistry
- Microbiology
- Serology
- Haematology
- Blood bank
- Cytology
- Histology

**Responsibility of medical lab technician:-**

- Prevention and control of laboratory accidents.
- Collecting blood or specimen sample from patients.
- Cleaning equipment and maintaining sterile laboratory environment
- Patient sample and preparing them for test.
- Carry out sampling testing measuring, recording, and analysing.

**Lab safety rules:-**

- Always wear an apron or protective clothing when working with chemicals.
- Always tie back loose hair
- Always wear goggles or safety glasses to prevent getting materials in your eyes.
- Always read the labels on chemical and read all warning.
- Never play around during experiment.
- Always wash your hands after handling lab materials.

# BIOCHEMISTRY

## INTRODUCTION TO CLINICAL BIOCHEMISTRY:-

Clinical biochemistry is one of the most rapidly advancing areas of a clinical Laboratory which deals with various biochemical parameters of the body.

The human body is a complex structure and many chemical reactions take place In The human body. Clinical biochemistry involves analytical measurement of Different chemical constituents of the body fluids like serum, plasma, urine CSF Etc. at the molecular level.

## PRINCIPLE OF FIRST AID:-

1) Preserve life

- Air way
- Breathing
- Circulation

2) Prevent deterioration

- Stop bleeding
- Treat shock
- Treat other injuries

3) Promote recovery

- Reassure
- Relive pain
- Handle with care
- Protect from harm

## Recommended contains of laboratory first aid box include:-

- Sterile in medicated dressing to cover wound
- Absorbent cotton wool
- Triangular and roll bandages

- Sterilize adhesive water proof dressing in a variety of size
- Sterile eye pads
- Roll of adhesive tape
- Scissors
- Sodium bicarbonate powder
- Boric acid
- 5% acetic acid

## BIO – WASTE MANAGEMENT ENVIRONMENTAL HEALTH AND SOCITY:-

An important part of solid waste generated in the medical industry requires special Handling & treatment prior to disposal in order to protect public health safety and The environment this particular type known as regulates medical waste (RMW).

Vacutainer tubes may contain additional substance that preserves blood for Processing in medical laboratory.

**Different names for medical waste:-**

1. Medical waste
2. Biochemical waste
3. Clinical waste
4. Biohezardous waste
5. Regulated medical waste
6. Infectious medical waste
7. Healthcare waste

- The list below the most common waste categorise as identified by the WHO.

**Yellow bag:-**

Infectious waste, bandage, gauze, cotton, or any other objects in contact with Body fluid, human body parts, placenta etc.

**Blue bag:-**

All things of glass bottles and broken glass.

**Black bag:-**

Discards medicines and cytotoxic drugs, radioactive substance.

**Green bag:-**

Recyclable waste, stationary waste, disposable paper, cups, domestic purpose Kitchen waste.

**Red Bag:-**

Microbiology & Biotechnology waste , body fluid, solid waste.

**Colour coding of bags for segregation:-**

Yellow - incineration treatment.

Red - autoclaving, microwaving, chemical treatment.

Blue - autoclaving, microwaving, chemical treatment.

Black - disposable in secured landfill.

**TREATMENT METHODS:-**

- Incineration

- Autoclaving

- Microwaving

- Chemical

- Biological

## CLEANING OF USED GLASSWARE FOR BIOCHEMICAL ANALYSIS PROCEDURE:-

- Used glassware given should be washed with water immediately after use.

- Soak in mild detergent solution for considerable period of time

- Wash thoroughly with running tap water

- Rinse with d/w

- Allowed to dry in hot air oven at 80c.

## ➤ CLINICALLY INSTRUMENTS:-

### Volumetric wares:-

- Volumetric wares are apparatus used for the measurement of liquid volume.

- They can be made from either glass or plastic wares such as pipettes, volumetric, flask, cylinders, burettes.

### Pipettes:-

- There are several types each having its own advantages & limitation pipettes are Designated as class "A" or "B" according to their accuracy.

- Class "A" pipettes are the most accurate and the tolerance limits are well.

- Class "B" pipettes are less accurate but quite satisfactory for most general Laboratory purpose.

### Volumetric pipettes:-

- Volumetric pipettes are calibrated to deliver a constant volume of liquid. The most Commonly used sizes are 1,5 and 10 ml capacities. Less frequently used sizes are those Which deliver 6, 8, 12 ml. They should be used when a high degree of accuracy is Desired. The pipettes is first rinsed several times with a little of the solution to be Used. Then filled to just above the mark.

**Graduated pipettes:-**

- Graduated pipettes are pipettes with various volume marked along the tube. They are used to measured and transfer an accurate volume of liquid from one container to another. Graduated pipettes are made from plastic or glass tubes that have a tapered tip. Along the body of the tube are lines indicating total volume.

**Micro pipettes:-**

- Micro pipettes are utilized in the laboratory to transfer small quantities of liquid.

They are commonly used in chemistry, biology, virology, immunology and serology Laboratories.

**Cylinders:-**

- A graduated cylinder is a piece of laboratory glassware used to measure the volume Of liquids. It is used to accurately measure the volume of chemical for use in reactions.

**Test tubes:-**

- Test tubes are widely used by chemist to handle chemicals especially for qualitative experiment and assays. Test tubes are convenient containers for heating small amounts of liquids or solids with a Bunsen burner or alcohol burner the tube is usually held by its neck with a clamp or tongs.

**Petri- dishes:-**

- Petri- dishes are flat glass or plastic containers which have a number of uses in the medical laboratory. They are used predominantly for the cultivation of organisms on solid media.

They are made with diameters of 5 to 14 cm to isolate and identify and study the characteristic of microorganisms.

**Cuvettes:-**

- A Cuvette is a kind of laboratory glassware usually a small tube of circular or square cross section sealed at one end made of plastic glass or optical grade quartz and designed to hold samples for spectroscopic experiment.

**Balance:-**

- Balance are widely used for weighing of various substances (Powder, crystals, others) in the laboratory.

Balances in medical laboratory two types

1. Rough balance
2. Analytical balance

**1) Rough balance :-**

- Two pan balances is a rough balance which has two copper pans supported by shafts it is used for to large amounts (up to several kilograms).

- When high degree of accuracy is not required.

**2) Analytical balance :-**

- Analytical and electronic balance (Single pan balance that use an electron magnetic force instead of weights) are the most popularly used balance in medical laboratory to provide a precision and accuracy for reagent and standard preparation.

- To weigh small quantities usually in (mg) range.

- Great accuracy is required.

**Centrifuge:-**

- Centrifuge is equipment that is used to separate solid matter from a liquid Suspension by means of centrifugal force.

- Basic components of centrifuges:-

- Central shaft:- It is part that rotates when spinning is effected manually

- Head :- It is part that holds the bucket and connected directly to the central Shaft or spindle.

- Bucket or tube :- This portions that hold test tubes containing a given sample to be spines.

**Types of centrifuge:-**

1. Micro centrifuge or serofuge

- They are used for spinning small tubes as in blood bank laboratories.

2. Medium size centrifuge

- This centrifuge used for urine specimens for microscopic analysis of urinary sediments.

3. Large centrifuge

- They are widely applied in bacteriology & medical chemistry laboratories. A centrifuge may have built in timer or may have to be timed with a watch.

**Hot air oven:-**

- Hot air ovens are instruments that are used for drying of chemicals and glassware's. They are also used for drying of chemicals and glassware's. They are also used for the Sterilization of various glassware's and metal instruments.

- They consist of double walls that are made of copper or steel. They are heated by circulation of hot air from gas burners between the metal walls.

**Water bath:-**

- Water bath is an instrument where water is heated and the set temperature is maintained a constant level. It is used to incubate liquid substance. When only a few samples in tubes require incubating.

Chemical test react best at a specific temperature many tests react room temperature & other requires a specific temperature.

**Incubator:-**

- Incubation at controlled temperature is required for bacteriological culture, blood transfusion, serology, haematology and medical chemistry test.

**Colorimeter:-**

- Colorimeter is an instrument used to measure the concentration of a substance in a sample by comparing the amount of light it absorbed with that absorbed by standard preparation containing a known amount of the substance being measured or a coloured derivative of it is produced this is measured in a colorimeter coloured solution absorbed light at given wavelength in the visible spectrum.

**Refraction**: - is defined as sudden change in the direction of the beam when the light

Passes from one medium to another with a different physical density.

**Reflection:** - is a condition where the beam returns back towards its source.

**Absorption:** - is a situation where some components of the light are retained or absorbed.

**Flame photometry:-**

- Flame photometer is a spectral method in which excitation is caused by spraying a solution of the sample in a hot flame.

- A characteristic radiation is emitted in a flame by individual element and the emission intensity is proportional to the concentration of the element emits a radiant power with a specific wavelength. So using different filters elements in a mixture can be analyzed at different wavelength.

- Flame photometer is used for the determination of electrolytes in a given solution. It is most commonly used for the sodium & potassium ions in body fluids.

## MICROSCOPE:-

- Microscope is an important device that enables us to visualize minute's objects that cannot be seen by our naked eye.

**Major parts of microscope:-**

**Arm (stand):-**

- The basic frame of the microscopic to which the base body 7 stages are attached

**A Stage:-**

- The table of the microscope where the side or specimen is placed.

**A foot or base:-**

- Is the rectangular part up on which the whole instrument.

**Course adjustment:-**

- Adjustment is controlled by a pair of range knobs positioned one on each side of the body rotation of these knobs move the tube with its lenses.

**Fine adjustment:-**

- While low power objectives can be focused by the course adjustment high power Objectives require a fine adjustment.

**Objectives: -** Objectives are components that magnify the image of the specimen to form the primary image for most routine laboratory work. 10x, 40x and 100x objectives are adequate.

**Eyepiece:-**

- Eyepiece is the upper optical component that further magnifies the primary image and brings the light rays to a focus at the eye point. It consist of two lenses mounted at the correct distance. It is available in a range of magnification usually 4x, 6x,7x, 10x, 5x.

**Working principle of the microscope:-**

- A microscope is a magnifying instrument the magnified image of the object is first produced by a lens close to the object called the objective. This collects light from the specimen and form the primary image.

- The magnification of the objective multiplied by that of the eyepiece. Gives the total magnification of the image seen in the microscope.

**Types of microscope:-**

- **Compound microscope (simple):**

- Compound microscope is a light microscope which is routinely used in medical laboratory.

- **Phase contrast microscopy:-**

- Transparent microorganisms suspended in a fluid may be difficult and some time impossible to sees.
- Phase contrast is particularly useful for examining .unstained bacteria e.g. cholera.

- **Dark field microscope:-**

- It is an instrument used for lighting microorganism suspended in fluid, enabling their structure motility to be seen more clearly. It makes some living organisms visible.

- **Fluorescence microscope:-**

- Fluorescence microscope ultra violet light which has a very short wavelength and is not visible to the eye is used to illuminate organisms, cells, or particles which have bee previously stained with fluorescing dyes.

## Care & Cleaning microscopic:-

- Always carry a microscope using both hands.
- When not in use a microscope should be protected from dust, moist, direct sunlight and put in microscope case.
- At the end of each day`s work the surface lenses of the objectives, eyepiece and condenser should be cleaned using lens tissue.
- Never clean the lens of the objectives & eyepiece with alcohol.

## ➢ AUTOMATION:-

### Endpoint assay:-

- Endpoint reactions are especially suitable for chemical reaction which is the complete in a relatively short time and they produce one product for each molecule of analyte.

### Kinetic assay:-

- Enzyme activity is mostly determine by a rate reaction rather than an endpoint reaction. In such cases determine of the enzyme concentration is based on how fast a fixed amount of substrate is converted to product.

**Types of errors:-**

- Two major types of errors may occur in a laboratory.

**Random error:-**

- That arises due to in adequate control on the analytical variables patient identity, Sample labelling, sample collection, handling and transport etc.

**Systemic error:-**

- That occur due to in adequate control on analytical variables e.g. Due to error in calibration, unstable calibration material, unstable reagent blank etc.

**Types of analyzers:-**

**Semi – auto analyzer:-**

- It is a partial automation technique the samples and reagents are mixed and read manually calculation and reporting is done by the instrument.

**Fully auto analyzer:-**

- All the steps including pipetting and mixing of sample and reagent, incubation reading, calculation and reporting is done by the instrument.

**Batch analyzer:-**

- One parameter is estimate at a time enabling one batch of a specific test to be automatically conduct. The next parameter is estimate only after completion of one.

**Random access auto analyzer:-**

- These analyzer can store more than one reagent, samples are placed in the machine and the computer is programmed to carry out any number of selected tests on each sample priority can be given to test any sample or any specific order they can perform single test, profile pattern or emergency test.

**Electrolyte analyzer:-**

- Electrolyte analyzer are the latest automated instrument used for estimation of electrolytes such as sodium potassium etc. in place of flame photometer. The instrument uses ion selective electrodes and is based on the potentiometric method of ion measurement.

## ➤ TYPES OF SOLUTION:

**Percentage solution:-**

- A relationship of a quantity of solute to the quantity of solution multiplied by 100.

This is the most commonly used solution type in a medical laboratory percentage solution contains grams of solute per 100ml of solution.

**Saturated solution:-**

- A saturated solution is the solution that contain maximum amount of dissolve solute.

**Unsaturated solution:-**

- The solute concentration is the amount of solute or particles that are dissolve in solution.

**Molar solution:-**

- A molar solution is an aqueous solution that contain 1 mol (gram molecular weight) Of solute in 1 lit of the solution .molarity is the number of moles of solute per lit of solution, molar concentration is not same as molar solution.

**Normal solution:-**

- A solution that contains gram equivalents of a solute dissolved in the lit of the solution.

**Standard solution:-**

- Standard solution is a solution whose concentration is exactly known.

## ➢ QUALITY CONTROL:-

- Accuracy refers to the closeness of the estimate value to that of true value.

- Sensitivity is the ability of an analytical method to detect smallest quantities of the measured analyte.

- Analytical methods require calibration the process of relating the value indicated on the scale of the measuring device to the quantity required to be measured.

- Calibration is done using standard the solution refer to the known amount of a substance in a solution in which its concentration is expressed in terms of Moles or in weight per unit volume.

- Mean refers to the arithmetic average of set of values, a measure of central tendency of the distribution of a set of replicate result.

- **Standard deviation**: the average deviation between the individual scores in the distribution and the mean for the distribution.

**Standard**: Typical or average

- **Deviation**: Refers to the difference between an individual score and the average score for distribution.

- **Coefficient of variation**: The coefficient variation for a set of sample or population data expressed as a percent describes the standard deviation relative to the mean.

**Levey- jennings (L J) Chart**: Levey – Jennings chart is the most important control chart in laboratory quality control it can used for internal and external Quality control as well. It detects all kinds of analytical errors.

**Precision:-**

- It is completely independent of accuracy or truth and a method can be precise as determine by repeat analysis but the result can be inaccurate.

**Accuracy:-**

- Accuracy is concerned with the relationship of a set of results to the true value. This relationship is most conveniently measured by relating the mean of the replicate analysis to the true value.

- Precision does not mean accuracy because measurement may be highly precise but inaccurate due to a faulty instruments or technique.

**Sensitivity:-**

- Sensitivity can be defined in two ways, the first one is the ability of a diagnostic test to detect very small amounts of the analyte. The other is the ability of a test to detect truly infected individual.

**Specificity:-**

- It is the ability of a method to identify all samples which do not contain the substance being detected.

➢ **HANDLING AND STORAGE OF CHEMICAL IN A LABORATORY:-**

**Types of chemical:-**

**Flammable: -** flammable is property of material relating how easily the material ignites or sustains a combustion reaction.

**Precaution:-**

- Ensure that all stored containers are in good condition closed and properly labelled.
- Appropriate training and available information.
- Always wear the correct personal protective equipment.
- Never use flammable chemicals near potential ignition sources.
- Keep flammable materials close to where they will be used.

## Corrosive chemicals:-

- Corrosive material is a highly reactive substance that cause obvious damage to living tissue .corrosives act either directly by chemically destroying the part or indirectly by causing inflammation acids and bases are common corrosive materials corrosive chemicals are stored in amber coloured bottles at ground level.

## Precaution:-

- Eye protection.

- Skin protection.

- always add acids or bases to water.

- Store corrosive material away from heat / flames, oxidizer and water source.

Keep containers closed and ensure that manufactures labels and warning remain intact.

## Oxidizing chemical:-

- an oxidizing substance is one that produces heat or evolves oxygen in contact with other substances causing them to burn strongly or become explosive or spontaneously combustible.

E.g. - Hydrogen peroxide, nitric acid, ammonium nitrate, potassium dichromate.

## Precaution:-

- Avoid contact with flammable substances.

- wear the recommended protective equipment and clothing.

- Store away from of heat and ignition.

- Keep away from combustible materials.

**Explosive chemical:-**

- an explosion is very rapid chemical reaction that produces heat and gaseous products.

- Explosions produce a large amount of heat in a very short time period.

- Molecular fragmentation converts the solid explosive material into an enormous number of gas molecules which will occupy a much greater volume further enhanced by the very high temperature of the explosion.

E.g. - Picric acid.

**Precaution:-**

- All wiring and electrical fitting should be properly and checked regularly.

- Different explosive should be stored separate boxes.

- Fire or smoking should be strictly prohibited within the radius of 50 M from the explosive store.

- Jerks or drops of explosive not be allowed to take place.

**Radioactive chemical:-**

- Spontaneous emission of radiation either directly from unstable atomic nuclei or as a consequence of a nuclear reaction.

- The radiation including alpha particles, electrons, and gamma rays, emitted by a radioactive substance.

- Radioactive contamination refers only to the presence of the unintended or undesirable radioactivity and gives no indication of the magnitude of hazard involve.

**Precaution:-**

- wear protective suits and gloves.

- Keep radioactive substance in a room enclosed by concrete.

- Use robotic arms to handle a strong radioactive.

- Shield of radioactive container has to be made of lead.

- do not eat and drink in radioactive lab.

- No smoking no open flames.

**Toxic chemicals:-**

- Toxic substance pose a wide range of health hazards such as irritation, Sensitization, carcinogenic .This may be due to the ability to damage.

- The genome or to the disruption of cellular metabolic process. E.g. potassium cyanide.

**Precaution:-**

- Prevent the release of toxic vapours, dust, gases into the workplace.

- Wear appropriate personal protective equipment.

- to avoid exposure or contact with contaminated.

# BIOCHEMICAL TEST

## ➢ LIVER FUNCTION TEST

## BILIRUBIN:-

## INDICATION:-

- Bilirubin test used to help determine the cause of jaundice or help diagnose condition such as liver disease, haemolytic anaemia and blockage of the bile duct.

## PHYSIOLOGY:-

- Bilirubin is a tetrapyrole and breakdown product of heme catabolism.

- Bilirubin is created by the activity of biliverdin reductase on biliverdin. A green tetrapyrolic bile pigment that is also product of heme catabolism Bilirubin when oxidized reverts to became biliverdin, once again this cycle in addition. Bilirubin main physiologic role is as cellular antioxidant.

## INTERPRETATION:-

### Unconjugated (indirect) Bilirubin

This like Bilirubin created from RBC breakdown it travels in the blood to the liver. Cirrhosis, blood transfusion, haemolytic anaemia, gallstones, alcoholic disease.

### Conjugated (Direct) Bilirubin

This is the Bilirubin once it reaches the liver and undergoes a chemical change it moves to the intestines before being removed through your stool. Obstruction of the biliary, various types of hepatitis.

## ➢ ALKALINE PHOSPHATASE

**INDICATION:-**

- Elevated levels may be indication of condition such as various types of cancer, bone disease, liver disease, hepatitis, blood disorders, and pancreas.

**PHYSIOLOGICAL:-**

Alkaline phosphatise in main sources liver, bone, placenta & intestine infancy & childhood from growing bone, pregnancy due to placenta isoenzme.

**INTERPRITATION:-**

Paget's disease, rickets, carcinoma Prehepatic – normal, toxic hepatic – moderate hepatic, hepatobiliary – increase, Post hepatic – very high.

## ➢ ALT / SGPT / (Serum Glutamic Pyruvic Transaminase )

**INDICATION:-**

- primarily used to diagnose liver disease.

- monitor treatment for hepatitis.

- High concentration in liver and low concentration in heart muscle and kidney.

- ALT also differentiates between haemolytic jaundice and jaundice due to liver disease.

**PHYSIOLOGY:-**

- Homodimeric Cytoplasmic pyridoxal phosphate- dependent (Co enzyme).

- found in plasma and various body tissues greatest abundance in the liver.

- Lesser extent in kidneys, heart, brain,

- ALT catalyze the transfer of an amino group from L- alanine to alpha – ketoglutarate

- The products of this reversible transamination reaction being pyruvate & L- glutamate

## INTERPRETATION:-

- Liver damage due to hepatitis / cirrhosis.

- Exposure to carbon tetrachloride.

- Intake of certain medication, myopathy.

 - Lead poisoning, bile duct problems, diabetes, congestive heart failure.

### ➤ AST / SGOT (Serum Glutamic Oxaloacetic Transaminase)

- When a person shows symptoms of liver disease – fatigue weakness, nausea, vomiting abdominal pain or swelling, jaundice.

## PHYSIOLOGY:-

- Aspartate transaminase catalyzes the interconversion of aspartate and alpha- ketoglutarate to oxaloacetate and glutamate.

## INDICATION:-

- Acute viral hepatitis, cirrhosis, post heart attack.

- AST/ALT ratio is also increased after alcoholic hepatitis.

### ➤ GAMMA GLUTAMYL TRANSPEPTIDASE ( GGT) :-

## INDICATIONS:-

- Elevated in biliary obstruction, rickests, and osteosarcomas disease.

## PHYSIOLOGY:-

- It is found in blood stream and is especially of hepatic origin.

**INTERPRITATION:-**

- Higher value indicate bile duct obstruction cancer and necrosis of liver.

- Low level the liver is injured.

> **Lactate dehydrogenise (LDH):-**

**Indication:-**

- LDH is most often measured to check for tissue damage. LDH is in many body tissues especially the heart, liver, kidney, muscles, brain, lungs, blood cell. Other condition for which the test may be done include low red blood cell count (anaemia).

**Physiology:-**

- LDH is an enzyme that catalyzes the conversion of lactate to pyruvate. The end product of glycolysis into lactic acid. While the process of oxidative phosphorylation in the mitochondria. LDH maintain homeostasis in the absence of oxygen.

**Normal value: -** adults: 100 - 190 U/L

 Children: 60 - 170 U/L

**Interpretation:-**

Elevated levels of LDH can include

- Haemolytic anaemia
- Certain cancer
- Heart attack
- Stroke muscle injury
- Pancreatitis
- Liver disease

## ➢ AUSTRAILIAN ANTIGEN ( AA) :-

- AA is used to diagnose whether a patient is currently infected with the hepatitis B virus where hepatitis B persist longer than 6 month the infection becomes chronic & it becomes unlikely the patient will ever be completely cured.

## PHYSIOLOGY:-

- Structure & function the viral envelope of an enveloped virus has different surface proteins from the rest of virus which act as antigen these antigens are recognised by antibody proteins that bind specifically to one of these surface proteins.

## INTERPRITATION:-

- Indicates the person is infectious, found in high levels during acute & chronic infection, hepatitis means inflammation of the liver, less of appetite, fatigue, Nausea, vomiting, jaundice, discoloured urine & fecal matter.

## ➢ LIPID PROFILE

- A lipid panel is a blood test that measure lipids fat and fatty substance used source Of energy by your body lipid include cholesterol, triglyceride, HDL, LDL, they form Important constituent of nervous tissue.

## CHOLESTEROL:-

## INDICATION:-

- Cholesterol levels including diabetes mellitus type, obesity, alcohol & hypothyroidism, heart attack.

## PHYSIOLOGY:-

- Cholesterol it is also the precursor of the steroid hormones and bile acid.

- Cholesterol is insoluble in water it is transported in the blood plasma within lipoproteins.

- all the lipoproteins carry cholesterol.

**INTERPRITATION:-**

- Long standing elevation of serum cholesterol can lead to atherosclerosis.

- over period of decade's elevated cholesterol contributes to formation of atheromatous plaques in the arteries.

- Coronary heart disease.

➢ **TRYGLYCERIDE:-**

**INDICATION:-**

- Very high triglyceride levels may develop inflammation of the pancrease loss of appetite, vomiting.

**Physiology:-**

- Triglycerides are one of the types of fat transported in the blood stream.

- most of the body's fat is also stored in the tissues as triglycerides.

- Triglycerides are a mixture obtained from dietary sources and produced by the body as sources of energy.

**INTERPRITATION:-**

- Atherosclerosis, kidney disease, liver disease, obesity, alcoholism.

➢ **HIGH DENSITY LIPOPROTEIN (HDL):-**

**INDICATION:-**

- HDL as a risk factor for cholesterol.

- Atherogenesis.

**PHYSIOLOGY:-**

- HDL is known as good cholesterol because it transport cholesterol to your liver to be expelled from your body.

- HDL helps rid your body of excess cholesterol so it less likely to end up in your arteries.

**INTERPRITATION:-**

- Heart Attack, other heart disease.

> **VLDL (VERY LOW DENSITY LIPOPROTEIN)**

**INDICATION:-**

- VLDL contains the highest amount of triglyceride.

- VLDL this type of "BAD" cholesterol because it helps cholesterol build up on the wall of arteries.

**PHYSIOLOGY:-**

- VLDL is assembled in the liver form triglyceride, cholesterol & apolipoproteins.

- VLDL is converted in the blood stream to LDL and IDL (intermediate density lipoprotein).

- VLDL transport endogenous products.

**INTERPRITATION:-**

- VLDL thus further increase your risk of heart disease.

> **LDL (LOW DENSITY LIPOPROTEIN):-**

**INDICATION:-**

- LDL it takes cholesterol to your arteries where it may collect in artery walls, Too much cholesterol in your arteries may lead to a build up of plaque known as 'Atherosclerosis'.

**PHYSIOLOGY:-**

- LDL particles are formed as VLDL lipoprotein loses triglyceride through the action of lipoprotein lipase and they become smaller and dense containing a higher proportion of cholesterol ester.

- LDL are one of the five major groups of lipoprotein which transport all fat molecules around the body in the extracellular water.

**INTERPRITATION;-**

- This can increase the risk of blood clot in your arteries if a blood clot breaks away and block an artery in your heart or brain you may have a stroke or 'heart attack'.

> **ELECTROLYTES**

**- Sodium:-**

- Sodium low levels of blood sodium may be due to losing too much sodium most commonly from condition such as diarrhoea, vomiting, excessive sweating, Use of diuretics, kidney disease or low levels of cortisol, aldosterone and sex Hormones.

**PHYSIOLOGY:-**

- Sodium is the principal cation in the extra cellular fluid & its main function is related of blood volume maintain water balance & cell membrane potential it is also essential for acid – base balance & nerve conduction.

**INTERPRETATION:-**

- increased serum sodium hypernatremia.

- decreased total body water diabetes, insipidus.

- high levels – nausea, vomiting, ataxia, tremors.

➢ **POTASSIUM:-**

**INDICATION:-**

- Toxic elevation of serum potassium is observed in the case of patients with renal failure, treatment of hyperkalemia, cardiopulmonary.

**PHYSIOLOGY:-**

- Regulate intracellular osmorality, help for glycogen deposit in liver and skeletal Muscle, maintain normal cardiac rhythm maintain smooth muscle contraction.

**INTERPRETATION:-**

- Major caused of hyperkalemia include kidney disease or failure, acidosis, addisons`disease. Tachycardia and dilation of the heart with change in electrocardiogram.

➢ **Calcium:-**

**INDICATION:-**

- Pulse less electrical activity caused by severe hypocalcemia.

- Pancreatitis, hypervitaminosis.

**Physiology:-**

- Calcium absorption of small intestine.

- Play an important role in muscle relaxation and contraction present in higher amounts In bones along with phosphorous.

**INTERPRITATION:-**

Calcium test is ordered to monitor diseases of bone, kidney, and parathyroid gland and neurologic disorders. Decreased levels are seen in rickets and osteomalacia.

## ➢ CHLORIDE :-

**INDICATION**

- Cushing syndrome, chronic nephritis.

- Sometimes in over activity of the parathyroid glands.

**PHYSIOLOGY:-**

- Chloride is the major anion.

- Chloride plays a role in helping the body maintain a normal balance of fluids.

**INTERPRITATION:-**

- High chloride hyperchloremia.

- Lower levels indicates vomiting and diarrhoea.

- decrease activity of tubular reabsorption.

- Chloride is normally lost in the urine sweat and stomach secretion.

## ➢ BICARBONATE:-

**INDICATION:-**

- This test is usually performed respiratory alkalosis, metabolic acidosis, Hyperventilation.

**PHYSIOLOGY:-**

- The bicarbonate act as a buffer to maintain the normal levels of acidity in blood and other fluids in the body, acid – base balance.

**INTERPRITATION:-**

- Vomiting, salicylic poisoning, respiratory function, kidney disease Metabolic condition or other causes.

> **AMMONIA:-**

**INDICATION:-**

- impaired buffering action of kidney.

**PHYSIOLOGY:-**

- Ammonia arises from the hydrolysis of amino acid glutamine in kidney.

**INTERPRITATION:-**

- Increased levels indicate diabetic ketoacidosis and starvation.

- Decreased levels indicate carbohydrate rich diet.

> **KIDNEY FUNCTION TEST (RFT):-**

**Blood urea nitrogen (BUN):-**

**INDICATION:-**

- Elevated levels of urea are observed in pre- renal, renal, post- renal condition.

**Pre - renal:-** diabetes mellitus, dehydration, cardiac failure, severe burns.

**Renal condition:-** diseases of kidneys.

**Post - renal:-** enlargements of prostate stones in the urinary tract, tumour of the bladder.

**PHYSIOLOGY:-**

- It is the catabolic product of proteins and the excess is excreted in the kidneys.

**INTERPRITATION:-**

- Increased levels indicate heart and kidney damage.

- Decreased levels indicate malabsorption and low protein intake.

## ➢ UREA:-

High urea levels suggest poor kindly function this may be due to acute or chronic Kidney disease.

## INDICATION:-

- There are many things besides kidney disease that can affect urea levels such as decreased blood flow to the kidney as in congestive heart failure, shock, stress recent heart attack, severe burn, bleeding, kidney tumour, high protein diet.

## PHYSIOLOGY:-

- Low blood urea, very low protein diet as in malnutrition, severe liver damage inhibits urea cycle decreased urea formation and increase free ammonia leads to hepatic comma.

## ➢ CREATININE:-

- A creatinine blood test measures the levels of creatinine in the blood.

- Creatinine is a waste product that formas when creatinine breaks down.

- Creatinine levels are found in your muscle.

## PHYSIOLOGY:-

- Creatinine is synthesized primarily in the liver.

- Creatinine conversion to phosphocreatine is catalyzed by creatine kinase spontaneous formation of creatinine occurs during the reaction creatinine is removed from the blood chiefly by the kidneys primarily by glomerular filtration.

## INTERPRETATION:-

**Decreased:** - pregnancy, starvation, wasting, and disease. Corticosteroid, low protein intake dialysis.

**Increased:-**

- G.I bleeding, high protein diet, strenuous exercise, dehydration, renal failure shock, surgery, diabetic nephropathy.

## ➢ URIC ACID :-

**INDICATION:-**

- It is used in the treatment of chronic gout and hyperuricemia.

**PHYSIOLOGY:-**

- Uric acid is the end product of purine metabolism. The two purines found in RNA & DNA is adenine and guanine.

- Uric acid is filtered in the glomeruli & partially reabsorbed by the tubules and then it is excreted in urine.

**INTERPRETATION:-**

- The serum uric acid levels is often raised in gout the determination has diagnostic Value in differentiating gout from non gouty arthritis, uric acid, levels are also increased in renal failure, uremia and leukaemia.

## ➢ TOTAL PROTEINS:-

**INDICATION:-**

- Proteinuria, glomerularnephritis.

**PHYSIOLOGY:-**

- Proteins form very important constituent of the diet. They are mainly involved in body tissue and supplying energy.

- Its main sources are milk, eggs, liver, fish.

- Protein are denatured by HCL secreted by the parietal cells of the stomach.

- Protein in the plasma is made up of albumin & globulins.

- Nutritional status,

- Kidney disease

- Liver disease

## INTERPRITATION:-

- Extensive liver destruction, serum total proteins and albumin.

Decreased - renal disease, liver disease.

- Moderate Proteinuria - congestive heart failure and multiple myeloma,

Proteinuria - glomerularnephritis.

## ALBUMIN:-

- Albumin increase the dielectric constant of the medium and thus reduced zeta potential. Due to this effect the electrical repulsion between the red blood cell is less and the cells agglutinate.

- Mostly 22% bovine albumin is used as higher concentration can cause Rouleaux formation.

**Normal range: -** 3.4 to 5.4 g/dL

**Low levels:-**

- Malnutrition, Liver disease.

**High levels:-**

- Acute infection, burns, stress, heart attack.

## PROTHROMBIN TIME (PT):-

## INDICATION:-

- Blood clotting disorders.

## PHYSIOLOGY:-

- It measures the time taken for the blood to clot. It involves a lot of clotting factors from factor I to factor XIII.

## INTERPRITATION:-

- A prolonged prothrombin time indicate deficiency of vitamin K, Liver disease, deficiency of factors V, X, XII, fibrinogen and thrombin.

## ACTIVATED PARTIAL TIME (APPT):-

- The APPT assay is used to detect inherited & Acquired coagulation factor deficiency & quality of the intrinsic pathway to screen for heparin therapy.

- The assay will evaluated the function of fibrinogen prothrombin & factor V, VIII, X, XI, & XII.

## ➢ HORMONE TEST:-

## INDICATION:-

- The sex hormone test is useful in diagnosing a range of condition including fertility related issues and in diagnosing sex- hormone producing tumours.

## PHYSIOLOGY:-

- Sex hormone test is carried out to test the blood level of the major sex hormone Estrogen and progesterone in women and testosterone in men.

- Estrogen stimulates sexual maturity in females. Progesterone helps to maintain pregnancy.

- Testosterone stimulates male fertility and secondary sexual characters.

## INTERPRITATION:-

- **Estrogen low level** indicates ovarian failure, pituitary dysfunction or menopause.

- **High level** could indicate estrogens producing tumours or severe liver disease such as cirrhosis. In men it could indicate testicular tumours.

- **Progesterone low level** ovarian or pituitary gland dysfunction or pregnancy related problems.

- **High level** linked to ovulation pregnancy, ovarian cyst, adrenal gland disorders Or certain tumours.

**Testosterone low level** prostate cancer, orchiectomy (removal of the testes), Estrogen therapy, liver cirrhosis.

**High level** malignant tumours of adrenal gland and hyperthyroidism.

## ➢ FOLICAL STIMULATING HORMONE TEST (FSH):-

### INDICATION:-

- The test is usually carried out during certain time of menstrual cycle. The test is done to help diagnose for menopause, infertility, menstrual bleeding, and delayed puberty.

### PHYSIOLOGY:-

- **FSH** is a hormone released by the pituitary gland in the brain .it is responsible for stimulating the follicles of the ovaries to produce eggs in menstruating women.

- The levels of FSH vary throughout the menstruating cycle of a women and is known to peak just before the release of egg. In men it helps to stimulate the production of sperm.

### INTERPRITATION:-

- Higher values indicate hypopitutarism, genetic disorders like turner and knilfielters syndrome.

- Low values indicate disorders of pituitary and hypothalamus.

> **ADRENOCORTICOTROPHIC HORMONE ( ACTH) :-**

**INDICATION:-**

- The test is ordered to detect hormonal imbalances in the body, problems of the adrenal gland, multiple endocrines Neoplasia, cause of tumours in the body.

**PHYSIOLOGY:-**

- ACTH is a hormone released from the anterior pituitary gland in the brain, it is released by the hypothalamus called corticotrophin releasing hormone.

- The main function of ACTH is to regulate the production of cortisol.

- ACTH test is done to detect problems in the pituitary gland and the adrenal glands.

**INTERPRITATION:-**

- Higher than normal levels indicate the following:

- Addison's disease – low cortisol
- Congenital adrenal hyperplasia a condition seen at birth.
- Cushing's syndrome – causes tumours in pituitary gland, thyroid, pancreas
- Emotional or physical stress

- Lower than normal levels indicate the following:

- Damage to pituitary gland due to surgery
- Stroke, radiation, head injury, or a tumour
- Adrenal gland tumours or tumours in other parts of the body.

> **THYROID FUNCTION TEST :-**

**INDICATION:-**

- To rule out hypothyroidism in new born and adult

- To rule out hyperthyroidism

- To assess treatment for hypo/ hyperthyroidism

## PHYSIOLOGY:-

- Thyroid hormone tests are blood test that are done to assess the functioning of the thyroid gland.

- the thyroid is a butterfly – shaped gland that is located in front of the windpipe the help of iodine absorbed from food it makes two hormone thyroxin (T4) and iodothyronine (T3) which are stored in the thyroid and released to the body.

- Thyroid hormone T3 and T4 are required for the proper functioning of the brain.

## INTERPRITATION:-

- Higher than normal values could indicate the following:-

- Grave`s disease
- Thyroiditis
- Goiter
- Over consumption of thyroid medications

- Lower than normal values could indicate the following:-

- Thyroid disease
- Pituitary gland disease
- Thyroid gland damage through radiation /surgery

➢ **Prolectin: -**

**Indication:-**

- Indication for the Prolectin included infertility menstrual cycle disorders.

**Physiology:-**

Prolectin is polypeptide hormone produced in eosinophilic cell of the anterior pituitary.

- PRL is responsible of primarily initiating and sustaining and stimulation of breast development along with estrogens during pregnancy.

- Inhabitation of ovulation by decreasing secretion of LH and FSH during pregnancy.

- Regulation of immune system stimulating Tell function.

- Transporting fluid, NA, Cl, Ca, across epithelial intestinal membrane and promoting Na, K and water retention in the kidney.

**Normal range:** - males: 2 to 18 ng/mL

Females: 2 to 29 ng/mL

Pregnant females: 10 to 209 ng/mL

**Interpretation:-**

- Hypoprolactinaemia Causes

- Head injury
- Autoimmune disease
- Ovarian disease
- Abnormal spermatogenesis
- Hyperprolactinaemia causes:-
- Stress
- Pituitary gland tumours
- Infertility

## ➢ VITAMINS

- Vitamins are organic nutrients that are required in small quantities for a variety of biochemical function and which generally cannot be synthesized in the body and must be supplied by the diet.

**Classification:-**

**1) Water soluble :-**
   B complex
   C or Ascorbic acid
**2) Fat soluble :-**
   A or retinol
   D or cholecalciferol
   E or Tocopherol
   Vitamin K

➢ **VITAMIN – B1:-**

**INDICATION:-**

- Berry - berry

**PYHSIOLOGY:-**

- Vitamin B1 plays an important role in carbohydrate metabolism and nervous function.

**INTERPRITATION:-**

- Deficiency may be due to chronic alkalosis megaloblastic anaemia.

➢ **VITAMIN – E:-**

**INDICATIONS:-**

- Anaemia

**- PHYSIOLOGY:-**

- It is an antioxidant for unsaturated lipids.

- Vitamin E also plays a role in eye and neurological function and inhibition of platelet coagulation.

- Vitamin E also protects lipids and prevents the oxidation of polyunsaturated fatty acid.

**INTERPRITATION:-**

- Deficiency leads to edema, haemolytic anaemia, ataxia, myopathies, and red blood cell destruction, retinopathy.

## ➢ VITAMIN – B6:-

**INDICATION:-**

- Dermatitis hypochromic anemia, Depression, Atherosclerosis, Early stroke.

**PHYSIOLOGY:-**

- It plays an important role in glycogen metabolism.

**INTERPRITATION:-**

- Early myocardial infarction, peripheral neuropathy, generalized seizures, Haematological manifestations.

## ➢ VITAMIN –K

**INDICATION:-**

- Impaired blood clotting, inflammatory bowel diseases.

**PHYSIOLOGY:-**

- Promoted blood clotting, vascular biology, bone metabolism.

Lipid soluble vitamin –k.

- Vitamin k is stored in the fatty tissue of the human body.

**INTERPRITATION:-**

- Liver damage or disease, cystic fibrosis or inflammatory bowel disease.

- Anaemia bruising, menstrual bleeding in women.

- Haemolytic disease.

## ➢ VITAMIN B12 :-

- Vitamin B12 also called cobalamine is a water soluble vitamin. The normal functional of the brain and nervous system and for the formation of blood.

- Vitamin B12 is important for metabolism the formation of red blood cell and the maintenance of the central nervous system which includes the brain and spinal cord.

**Absorption of B12:-**

- Gastric acid and pepsin release the vitamin from protein binding in food and make it available to bind to Vitamin B12 deficiency include:

- Fatigue
- Depression
- Muscle pain
- Memory loss
- Diarrhoea
- Menstrual problems
- Weight loss

## ➢ VITAMIN – D:-

**INDICATION:-**

- Osteomalacia

**PHYSIOLOGY:-**

- Vitamin –D regulates minerals such as calcium and phosphorus found in the body and plays an important role in maintaining proper bone structure.

- Vitamin –D has a significant role in calcium homeostasis and metabolism.

- Vitamin –D levels can be easily restored through sun exposure.

**INTERPRITATION:-**

- Rickets, osteomalacia.

> **FOLIC ACID :-**

**INDICATION:-**

- Anaemia

**PHYSILOGY:-**

- It plays an important role in nucleic acid & amino acid biosynthesis.

**INTERPRITATION:-**

- Deficiency is due to poor absorption and insufficient dietary intake.

> **TUMOUR MARKER**

**ONCOFETAL ANTIGENS:-**

- **ALPHA – FETOPROTEIN ( AFP )**
- **CARCINO EMBRYONIC ANTIGEN ( CEA )**
- **SQUAMOUS CELL CARSINOMA ( SSC )**

**ALPHA – FETOPROTIEN (AFP):-**

- It is marker for heptocellular & germ cell carcinoma, they indicative control of pregnancy.

- AFP also associated with hepatitis and cirrhosis of liver.

- High level are indicative of cancer.

**CARCINO EMBRYONIC ANTIGEN (CEA):-**

- CEA is a marker for colorectal, gastrointestinal, lung & breast carcinoma.

- persistently elevated level suggest the presence of colon cancer.

- CEA is also useful in monitoring breast, gastric & pancreatic carcinoma.

**Squamous cells carcinoma (SSC):-**

- SCC antigen is including those of the cervix, lung, skin, head, neck, ovaries, Urogenital tract and digestive tract.

## CARBOHYDRATE AS TUMOR MARKERS:-

### CA 15- 3:-

- CA 15- 3 is marker for breast carcinoma.

- Elevated levels of CA 15- 3 are also found in other malignancies including pancreatic, Lung, ovarian.

### CA - 125:-

- Is marker for ovarian & endometrial carcinomas.

- It is also found in breast, gastrointestinal tumours.

## PROSTATE SPECIFIC ANTIGEN (PSA):-

- Prostate cancer is the leading cancer in older man.

- PSA in prostatic tissue & not present in other tissue.

- PSA determination are used for early detection of prostate cancer & also for monitoring treatment.

## CK- MB (CREATINE KINASE MB):-

- **CK- MB** is a sensitive marker for myocardial injury.

- Widely distributed in tissue with highest activity in skeletal muscle, heart muscle, Brain tissue.

- Higher levels are due to myocardial breakdown and central nervous system shock.

- Myocardial infraction, skeletal muscle disorders.

**CPK (CREATINE PHOSPHOKINASE):-**

- CPK activity is highest in brain, heart muscle.

- elevated levels poly myositis, motor – neuron disorders, acute cerebro vascular accidents.

**ACID PHOSPHATASE (ACP):-**

**INDICATION:-**

- An Acid phosphate test is mostly advice to evaluate the spread of prostate cancer increased level of ACP is also seen in cases of hyperthyroidism, gauchaer`s disease and some blood cell disease.

- The test may also be ordered to analyze dysfunction in the heart, liver, or other organs.

- ACP is also ordered during rape investigation as the levels of the enzyme are very high in the semen.

**PHYSIOLOGY:-**

- ACP is primarily found in the prostate gland. It is also present in the spleen, Liver, blood cells, and bone marrow. If any of the organs or tissues is not functioning in the proper manner they tend to release ACP in to the blood strem.

**INTERPRITATION:-**

- High level indicates:-

- Prostate cancer
- Kidney disease
- Paget`s disease – A Condition that makes bones thick and soft
- Anaemia – low red blood cell count
- Prostatitis – inflammation of prostate
- Thrombophlebitis – inflammation and small blood clots in a vein mostly in the leg

- Multiple myeloma – malignancy affecting the plasma cells of the bone marrow

> **METABOLIC SCREENING**

**GLYCOSYLATED HAEMOGLOBIN:-**

**INDICATION:-**

- Persistence of hyperglycemia.

**PHYSIOLOGY:-**

- Glucose combines with haemoglobin to form glycated haemoglobin. The levels indicate at any point of time the average blood glucose levels for the past 3 to 4 month.

**INTERPRITATION:-**

- High levels have been reported in iron deficiency anaemia, Hyperglycemias.

**DIABETES MELLITUS:-**

**INDICATION:-**

- Impaired glucose tolerance.

**PHYSIOLOGY:-**

- It exists in 4 forms as type 1 (IDDM) or type 2 (NIDDM), other specific type of diabetes and gestational diabetes mellitus.

- Type - 1 is characterised by self destruction of pancreatic cells resulting in absolute deficiency of insulin.

- Type- 2 is characterised by individual's resistance to insulin and it is the majority.

**INTERPRITATION:-**

- Hyperglycemia impaired fasting blood glucose.

**GLUCOSE - 6- PHOSPHATE DEHYDROGENASE (G6PD):-**

**INDICATION:-**

- This test is used to detect drug sensitive population of red cells due to G- 6-PD Deficiency to determine the cause of hemolysis.

**PHYSIOLOGY:-**

- G- 6- PD deficiency due to the ingestion of above mentioned drugs, oxidation of haemoglobin takes place with the formation of methemoglobin followed by Heinz body formation.

**INTERPRITATION:-**

- G- 6- PD deficient hemolysis may also be secondary to acute bacterial or viral infection and metabolic disorders such as acidosis.

# HEAMATOLOGY

## INTRODUCTION OF HEMATOLOGY

- Hematology the study of blood cells and coagulation included in its concern are analysis of the concentration, structure and function of cells in blood.

- Blood is circulating tissue composed of fluid plasma and cells. It is composed of different kinds of cells these formed elements of the blood constituent about 45% of whole blood. The other 55% is blood plasma a fluid that is the blood liquid medium, appearing yellow in colour.

- The normal PH of blood 7.40. A blood volume of about 5 litters of which 2.7- 3 litters are plasma in human body.

➢ **Hemoglobin:-**

- Hemoglobin is the protein molecule in red blood cells that carries oxygen from the lungs to the body`s tissues and returns carbon dioxide from the tissues back to the Lungs.

- Hemoglobin is made up of four protein molecules that are connect together.

- **Normal value:-** children - 11 to 13 gm/dL

Adult males - 14 to 18 gm/dL

Adult women - 12 to 15 gm/dL

➢ **HEMATOPOITIC SYSTEM OF THE BODY**

- Hematopoiesis is **Production, development, maturation** of cellular elements of bloods.

- **Hem = blood, poiesis = synthesis** it consist of production of erythrocytes (Erythropoiesis), leukocytes (leucopoiesis), thromobocytes (hrombocytopoiesis).

**Normal sites for poises**

- Fetus less than 2 month : Yolk sac

- 2 to 7 month : Liver and spleen (partially)

- After 3 month : Bone marrow

- Full term infant : Bone marrow

- Children and the adults : Bone marrow

- Development of blood cells takes place through 3 stages.

1) Multiplication of precursor cells
2) Structural and functional maturation
3) Release in to the peripheral circulation

## ➢ ERYTHROPOIESIS

- Erythropoiesis is the process which produces red blood cells .it is stimulated by decreased O2 in circulation, which is detected by the kidneys which then secrete the hormone erythropoietin.

**Leukopoiesis:-**

- Leucopoiesis is the production of white blood cells .It has three independent series which lead to formation of **Granulocytes, lymphocytes and monocytes**.

- The granulocytes are formed in the bone marrow and the process of maturation is divided into six stages.

**- Development of Neutrophil: -**

- Neutrophil are most abundant type of granulocytes. They form an essential part of the innate immune system.

- They are formed from stem cells in the bone marrow.

- **Development of Lymphocytes:-**

- Morphologically the lymphocytes are divided as small lymphocytes and large lymphocytes.

- All lymphocytes originate during this process from a common lymphoid progenitor before differentiating into their distinct lymphocyte types.

- **Development of Eosinophil:-**

- Eosinophils develop from bone marrow progenitor cell. Which in turn develops in to myelocyte and then in to mature Eosinophil.

- **Development of Monocytes:-**

- Monocytes develop from myelo – monocytic stem cells in the bone marrow. Then go in to blood where they circulated for a few days in order to then migrate in to tissues in the tissue they further mature in to macrophages.

- **Development of Basophil:-**

- Basophil develop from precursor cells in the bone marrow that expand in number in response to growth factors. Once mature basophils exit the bone marrow and enter the periphery.

➤ **FUNCTION OF ERYTHROPOIETIN:-**

- Erythropoietin increase RBC production in 3 ways;

- Promotes pronormoblasts production
- Shortens the transition time through the normoblast stage
- Promotes the early release of reticulocytes.

➤ **THROMBOPOIESIS:-**

- Thrombocytes are ligation of the cytoplasm from megakaryocytes. A single megakaryocyte can give rise to thousand of Thrombocytes. The term thrombocytopoiesis is sometime used to emphasize the cellular nature.

> ## FUNCTIONAL CLASIFICATION & COLOUR CODES

Red cap: - this vacutainers are separate serum .these are free additive vacutainers used for test for chemistry.

Purple cap: - this vacutainers are separate plasma. This tube used for whole blood.

Green cap: - this vacutainers are separate plasma. This tube contain sodium heparin, lithium heparin.

Light blue: - this vacutainers are separate plasma. These tubes contain sodium citrate in measure amount & useful in blood coagulation assays.

Yellow cap: - they utilized for serum testing they contain rapid clot activator they used for serum immunology.

Light grey: - these tubes have sodium fluoride and potassium oxalate and are used for blood glucose determination.

> ## BLOOD COLLECTION

**Introduction:-**

- Three general procedures for obtaining blood are 1) skin puncture, 2) vein puncture

1)   Arterial puncture

**Skin puncture / capillary blood collection:-**

- Capillary blood is frequently used when only small quantities of blood are required in case of severe burns in extreme obesity where locating the veins could be a Problem.

**Advantages of capillary blood:**

- It is obtained with easy.

- It is less painful

- It is ideal for peripheral blood smears

- Disadvantages of capillary blood:

- Less amount of blood can be obtained.

- Additional and repeated tests cannot be done

- Blood obtained by skin puncture hemolysis easily

**Venous blood collection:-**

- Venous blood is the specimen of choice for most routine laboratory tests. The blood is obtained by direct puncture to a vein most often located in the antecubital area Of the arm or back of the hand.

- The three main veins in the forearm 1) cephalic 2) Median cephalic 3) Median basilic.

**Advantages of venous blood:**

- By providing sufficient amount of blood it allow various tests to be separated in case of accident or breakage or for the all important checking of doughtful result.

- The specimen Plasma and serum may be frozen for future reference.

Disadvantages of venous blood:

- It is a lengthy procedure that requires more preparation than the capillary method.

- It is technically difficult in children, obese individuals and in patients in shock.

**Arterial puncture:-**

- Arterial blood is used to measure oxygen and carbon dioxide and to measure PH Arterial blood gases (ABG).

- The blood gas measurements are critical in assessment of oxygenation problems in patients. With pneumonia, pulmonary embolism arterial punctures are technically more difficult to perform than venous punctures.

**Prevention of hemolysis**

- Make sure the syringe needle and test tubes are dry and free from detergent as trace of water or detergent cause hemolysis

 - use smooth good quality sharp needle

- Transfer the blood from the syringe by gently ejecting down the side of the tube mix blood with anticoagulant by gently inversion not by shaking.

- Tourniquet should not be too tight and should be released before blood is aspirate.

- If examination is to be delayed beyond 1- 3 hrs do not allow the sample to stand unsealed or at room temperature.

## ➢ IMPROVED NEUBAUER CHAMBER

- In this the triple lines which dividing the central large square are very much closer to each other. The central ruled area is divided into 25 large squares. These squares are subdivided to form 16 smaller squares each with an area of 1/400 of 1.5 sq mm. The depth of improved Neubauer chamber is same i.e. 0.1mm.

**Old Neubauer chamber:-**

- In this the central platform is set 0.1mm below the level of the two side which giving the chamber a depth of 0.1mm .the ruling covers an area of 9.0sq.mm divided into 16 larger squares by set of triple lines. These large squares are further subdivided into 16 small squares by single line.

# BLOOD BANK

> ## ➤ INTRODUCTION BLOOD

- The Goal of blood management is ensure the safe & efficient use of the many resource involved in the blood bank.

- Blood is collected from donors typed, separated into components, stored & prepared for transfusion to recipients.

- Recruitment of donors and maintenance of donor's record.

- Collection, preservation & distribution of blood & Blood components.

- Laboratory procedures like testing for hepatitis B, hepatitis C, HIV, VDRL, for syphilis & Malaria parasite.

> ## ➤ BLOOD DONATION CRITERIA:-

- Criteria for blood donation;

- Age – 18 to 51 Years old.
- Weight - 50kg or above.
- Pulse rate – Normal.
- Blood pressure – Normal.
- The medical history normal.
- Unfit for blood donation infection e.g. HIV Syphilis, AIDS.
- Females pregnant for six month or above should not be selected as donors.
- Oral temperature should not exceed 37 c.

> ### ➤ Blood plasma:-

- When the formed elements are removed from blood a straw – coloured liquid called plasma is about 91.5% water and 8.5% solutes 7% proteins. These proteins play a role in maintaining proper blood osmotic pressure.

## ➤ STORAGE OF BLOOD AND BLOOD COMPONENTS

- Whole blood and red cell concentrate must always be stored between 2 to 6 C.

- The Temperature less than 2C can cause the red cells leading to haemolysis.

- Temperature more than 6 C can lead to over growth of non specific bacteria.

**Fresh frozen plasma (FFP)**

- FFP is usually transfused to restore or to maintain the clotting mechanism.

- FFP is prepared by removing plasma from a unit of blood within 6 hr of collection and snap freezing at - 70 C and storing at – 30 C.

**Platelets:-**

- Platelet are involved in the blood coagulation process & are given to treat or prevent bleeding.

- Platelet stored in large flat bags with as high surface to volume ratio and on agitators to facilitate oxygen diffusion.

- Platelets should be stored at 22 to 24 C in plasma under condition in which the PH is maintain at values above 6.8. A fall of PH of platelet concentrate due to lactate production from platelet glycolysis leads to loss of viability.

- Platelet stored 3 to 5 days depending on storage bag.

## ➤ ANTICOAGULANT PRESERVATIVE

- Trisodium citrate: - Rapid deterioration only 50% cells viable after 1 week.

- Acid citrate dextrose: - Strong viability for 28 days. 24 hr survival of 77%.

- Citrate phosphate dextrose (CPD):- Storage viability for 21 days .24 hr survival of 77%.

- Citrate phosphate dextrose – adenine (CPDA- 1):- Storage viability 35 days .improved storage due to adenine which maintains high ATP level in the RBC.

## ➢ BLOOD TRANSFUSION REACTION

- Blood transfusion are most commonly done for blood components such as red blood cells, platelets, or plasma before a blood transfusion.

- Antibodies in the recipient`s blood can attack the donor blood if the two are not compatible. if the recipient`s immune system attacks the red blood cells of the donor it is called a hemolytic reaction.

- Another transfusion reaction type is the transfusion related acute lung injury (TRALI) this reaction usually occurs within six hours of receiving blood.

- A Transfusion reaction can also occur if a person receives too much blood this Is known as transfusion – associated circulatory overload (TACO) having too much blood can overload your heart.

- Iron overload due to too much iron from donor blood. This can damage your heart and liver.

- Transfusion reaction symptoms include:

- Back pain
- Dark urine
- Chills
- Fainting or dizziness
- Fever
- Skin flushing
- Shortness of breath
- Itching

## ➢ ABO BLOOD GROUP

- The A, B and O blood groups were first identified by immunologist Karl Landsteiner in 1901.

- The classification of human blood based n the inherited properties red boo cells as determine by the presence or absence of the antigens A and B which are carried on the surface of the red cells.

- Persons may thus have type – A type – B, O or type – AB blood.

- The other main grouping used is the Rhesus (Rh) system which is either negative or positive.

- Blood group is a combination of the ABO system and the Rh system.

**Blood Group Antigens Present Antibodies present**

A Group A Antigen Anti – B

B Group B Antigen Anti – A

AB Group A & B Antigen No Antibody

O Group Neither Antigen Anti –A & Anti- B

## ➢ BOMBAY BLOOD GROUP

- **It is also called the HH group** .the peculiarity is that they do not express the H antigen. As a result they cannot form A antigens or B antigens on their red blood cells.

- Thus they can donate blood to anybody with ABO grouping but can receive blood  only from Bombay blood group.

- This can detect test is conducted with reagent called H lacten.

- The maternal production of anti – H during pregnancy might cause hemolytic disease in a fetus.

## ➤ CROSS MATCH

- Cross matching is a procedure performed prior to a blood transfusion to determine whether donor blood is compatible or incompatible with recipient blood.

- Compatibility is determined through matching of different blood group systems.

- The cross match is routinely used as the final step of pretransfusion compatibility testing. The purposes of compatibility testing are to detect irregular antibodies errors ABO groping and clerical errors in patient.

**- Major cross match:-**

- Major cross match this is the important cross match comparing donor red blood cell to recipient serum .antibodies in recipient serum against donor red blood cells.

**- Minor cross match:-**

- Minor cross match in contrast to the major cross match comparing donor red blood cells recipient serum .the donor serum with the recipient red cells.

## ➤ COOMBS TEST:-

- A Coombs test also known as antiglobulin test or AGT is either two clinical blood test used in immune hematology and immunology.

- The two coomb's tests are the direct coomb test (DCT), indirect coomb's test (ICT).

- The DCT is used to test for autoimmune haemolytic anaemia. DCT is also detect the antibodies or complement proteins that are bound to the surface of RBC.

- A Blood sample is taken and the RBCs are washed and then incubated with anti –human globulin (also known as coomb's reagent). If this produces agglutination of RBCs.

- The direct coomb's test is positive indication that antibodies are bound to the Surface of RBC.

**INDIRECT COOMBS TEST:-**

- ICT is used in prenatal testing of pregnant women and in testing blood prior to a blood transfusion.

- It detects antibodies against RBCs that are present unbound in the patient's serum. serum is extracted from the blood sample taken from patient then the serum incubated with RBCs of known antigenicity finally anti- human globulin is added .if agglutination occurs the direct coomb's test is positive.

> **DU**

- This test for a weak expression of the D antigen. Red blood cells that react weakly or not at all in direct agglutination test with anti- D may react with anti- D by the indirect antiglobulin test (IAT).

- The red cells are washed to remove unbound antibody (IgG – Anti- D) then tested with anti IgG.

# ANAEMIA

> **IRON DEFICIENCY ANEMIA :-**

- The most common form of anemia is iron deficiency anemia which is usually due to chronic blood loss caused by excessive menstruation.

- Increased demands for iron such as foetal growth in pregnancy and children rapid growth.

- The most common symptoms of chronic anaemia include tiredness, weakness, shortness of breath and sometimes a fast heartbeat.

- The tongue may also become smooth, shiny and inflamed this called glossitis .The symptoms of the cause of the iron deficiency.

> **APLASTIC ANEMIA:-**

- Aplastic anemia is a blood disorder in which the body`s bone marrow doesn`t make enough new blood cells.

- This may result in a number of health problems including arrhythmias, an enlarged heart, heart failure, infections and bleeding.

- Damage to the bone marrow `s stem cells causes' Aplastic anaemia.

- A number of acquired diseases, condition, and factors can cause Aplastic anemia including;

- Infectious diseases such as hepatitis, Epstein – Barr virus, cytomegalovirus and HIV.

- Autoimmune disorders such as lupus and rheumatoid arthritis.

- The most common symptoms of Aplastic anemia are;

- Fatigue
- Shortness of breath
- Dizziness
- Headache

- Coldness in your hands or feet
- Chest pains

## ➤ HAEMOLYTIC ANEMIA:-

- Haemolytic anemia is a condition in which red blood cells are destroyed and removed from the blood stream.

- Haemolytic anaemia can lead to various health problems such as fatigue, pain, Enlarged heart or heart failure.

- inherited haemolytic anemias include

- Immune haemolytic anemia
- Thalassaemia
- G6PD deficiency
- Certain infection and substance can also damage red blood cells and lead to haemolytic anemia.
- Sickle cell anemia

- **Symptoms of haemolytic anemia:-**

- Jaundice

- Pain in the upper abdomen

- A severe reaction to a blood transfusion

## ➤ THALASSEMIA:-

- Thalassaemia are inherited blood disorders. The two major types of Thalassaemia are alpha **and** beta **Thalassaemia. And major Thalassaemia.**

- **Alpha Thalassaemia:-**

- This type of Thalassaemia also has two serious types; haemoglobin H disease and hydrops fetalis.

- **Haemoglobin H; (HbH)** – disease is a form of alpha Thalassaemia in which moderately severe anemia develops due to reduced formation of alpha globin chains. In this condition as in the other forms of Thalassaemia there is an imbalance of globin chains. This disease can lead to bone tissues. The cheeks, forehead, all overgrow additionally haemoglobin H disease can cause:

- Jaundice
- An extremely enlarged spleen

- **Hydrops fetalis** is an extremely severe form of Thalassaemia that occurs before birth.

- This condition develops when all four alpha globin genes are altered or missing.

**Beta Thalassaemia: -** beta Thalassaemia occurs when your body can`t produce beta globin.

- Beta Thalassaemia include:-

- Fatigue, weakness, shortness of breath
- Irritability
- Slow growth
- A swollen abdomen
- Dark urine

## SICKLE CELL ANEMIA:-

- Sickle cell anemia is a serious disease in which the body makes sickle – shaped red blood cells.

- Sickle cells contain abnormal haemoglobin that causes the cells to have a sickle shape which don`t move easily through the blood vessels. They are stiff and sticky and tend to form clumps.

- The clumps of sickle cells block blood flow in the blood vessels that lead to the limbs and organs. Blocked blood vessels can cause pain, serious infection and organ damage.

- Sickle cell anemia is an inherited, lifelong disease.

- Signs and symptoms:-

- Fatigue
- Dizziness
- Pale skin
- Chest pain
- Shortness of breath
- Sudden pain through the body is a common symptom of sickle cell anemia,this pain is called a "Sickle cell crisis" and often affects the bones, lungs, abdomen, and joints.

## ➢ PERNICIOUS ANEMIA:-

- Pernicious anemia is a condition in which the body can`t make enough healthy red blood cells because it doesn`t have enough vitamin B12.

- The vitamin B12 deficiency may also have some serious symptoms such as:

- Nerve damage
- Neurological problems such as confusion, depression and memory loss
- The digestive tract include nausea and vomiting, heart burn, abdomen blotting and gas, weight loss, loss of appetite
- An enlarged liver
- Infants who have vitamin B12 deficiency may have poor reflexes or unusual movement such as face tremors.

## ➢ FANCONI ANEMIA:-

- Fanconi anemia or FA is a rare inherited blood disorder that leads to bone marrow failure. FA is a type of Aplastic anemia.

- FA can also cause your bone marrow to make many abnormal blood cells. This can lead to serious health problems such as leukemia.

- FA is a blood disorder but it can also affect many of the body's organ, tissues and systems.

- Signs and symptoms;-

-   Anemia
-   Bone marrow failure
-   Developmental or eating problems

- The four main types of treatment for FA are:

-   Blood and marrow stem cell transplant
-   Androgen therapy
-   Synthetic growth factors
-   Gene therapy

# HAEMATOLOGY TEST

## ➢ PREPARATION OF THIN BLOOD FILMS

- Three methods of making films are described.

 1. Wedge method

2. Cover glass method

3. Spinner method

- Preparation of blood films on glass slide has the following advantages -

- Slides are not easily broken

- Slide are easier to label

- When large number of films are to be dealt with slides will be found much easier handle.

## 1. Wedge method (Two – slide method):-

- A small drop of blood is placed in the center line of a slide about 1- 2 cm from one end. Another slide the spreading slide placed in front of the drop of blood at an angle of 30 to the slide and then is moved back to make contact with the drop.

- The drop will spread out quickly along the line of contact of the spreader with the slide once the blood has spread completely the spreader is moved forward smoothly and with a moderate speed.

- The drop should be of such size that the film is 3- 4 cm in length. It is essential that the slide used as a spreader have a smooth edge narrower in breadth. If the edges of the spreader are rough films with ragged tails will result and gross qualitative irregularity in the distribution of cells will be the rule.

- The bigger leucocytes will accumulate in the margins .thickness and length of the film are affected by speed of spreading and the angle at which the spreader slide is held.

- Once the slide is dry the name of the patient and date is written on the head of the film using a lead pencil or graphite and then fix it.

**Cover glass method:-**

- Take a clean cover glass

- Touch it on the drop of a blood

- place it on another similar cover glass in cross wise direction with side containing drop of blood facing down.

- pull the cover glass quickly.

- dry it and stain it.

- The cover glass smear more time consuming and difficult technique and easily broken.

**Spinner method:-**

- Blood films that combine the advantages of easy handling of the wedge slide & uniform distribution of cells of the cover glass reparation.

- Centrifuge spins slide briefly at 5000 rpm can be used with automated differential analyzer.

## ➢ PREPARATION OF THICK BLOOD SMEAR

- These are widely used in the diagnose of haemoparasites, particularly malarial parasites. Generally the blood films should be made about 10 times thickness of normal smears .

- Place a drop of blood on a clean slide and spread it with the corner of another slide until the printed matter is just visible through the smear.

- allow to air dry and label the slide properly

## ➢ COMPLETE BLOOD COUNT (CBC)

- The CBC is one of the most commonly blood test.

- The major cells in the blood are white blood cell (WBC), Red blood cells (RBC) and platelets. Each of these types of cells carries out specific and important function.

- The other components represent additional information about these cells including their size, colour, function, and maturity.

- Hematocrit (Hct)

- Hemoglobin (Hbg)

- Mean corpuscular volume (MCV)

- Mean corpuscular haemoglobin (MCH)

- Mean corpuscular haemoglobin concentration (MCHC)

- Red Cell distribution width (RDW)

- Mean Platelet volume (MPV)

## HEMOGLOBIN (Hbg):-

- Hbg measure the amount of the haemoglobin molecule in a volume of blood.

- Hemoglobin delivers oxygen from the lungs to the entire body then it returns to the lungs with carbon dioxide which we exhale.

- Low levels of haemoglobin may indicate anemia.

Normal range - 13.8 to 15.1 g/dl for men

 12.1 to 14.3 g/dl for women

**WBC (WHITE BLOOD CELL):-**

- WBC is important part of your body `s immune system they are responsible for protecting your body against infection.

- It may indicate leukemia which can increase in the number of WBC or other hand too few WBC could be caused by certain medication or health disorders.

- Normal range - 4,300 to 10,800 cmm

**Red blood cell (RBC):-**

- RBC measure the number of red blood cells in a volume of blood.

- Normal range - 4.2 to 5.9 million cells per cmm

**HEMATOCRIT (Hct):-**

- Hct useful for diagnosing anemia, this test determine how much of the total blood volume in the body consist of red blood cells.

Normal range - 45% to 52% for men

 37% to 48% for women

**MEAN CORPUSCULAR VOLUME (MCV):-**

- MCV is the measurement of the average size or volume if a typical RBC in blood sample.

- Irregularities could indicate anemia and chronic fatigue syndrome.

- Normal range - 80 to 100 femtoliters

**MEAN CORPUSCULAR HEMOGLOBIN (MCH):-**

- MCH measure the amount of haemoglobin in an average RBC.

- High levels signal anemia, low levels indicate a nutritional deficiency.

- Normal range - 27 to 32 pg

## MEAN CORPUSCULAR HEMOGLOBIN CONCENTRATION (MCHC):-

- MCHC test the average concentration of hemoglobin in a specific amount of RBC

- Low levels are hypochromic anemia

- High levels are spherocytosis

- Normal range - 32 to 36 %

## RED CELL DISTRIBUTION WIDTH (RDW):-

- Measure the variability in the size and shape of red blood cells Not the size of the cells liver disease, anemia, nutritional deficiencies

- Normal range - 11 to 15 %

## PLATELET COUNT:-

- Platelets are small portion of cells involved in blood clotting. Too many or too few platelets can affect clotting in different ways.

- 1, 50,000 to 4, 00,000 per cmm

## MEAN PLATELET VOLUME (MPV):-

- MPV measures and calculate the average size of platelets.

- These play a role in clotting.

- Higher MPV mean the platelets are larger which could risk for a heart attack or stroke.

- Lower MPV indicate smaller platelets risk for bleeding disorders.

- Normal range - 7.5 to 11.5 femtoliters

## WBC DIFFERENTIAL COUNT :-

- Five types of white blood cells:-

- Neutrophil - 40% to 60 %

- Lymphocytes - 20% to 40 %

- Monocytes - 2% to 8 %

- Eosinophils - 1 % to 4 %

- Basophiles - 0.5 % to 1%

- **Neutrophil** an **increase** in your blood may be caused by

- Acute stress

- Infection

- Rheumatoid arthritis

- Gout

- Pregnancy

- **Neutrophil decreased** in your blood may be caused by

- Anemia

- Bacterial infection

- Influenza or other viral illnesses

- Radiation exposure

- **Lymphocytes in increased** levels caused by

- Chronic infection

- Leukemia

- Viral infection such as mumps or measles

- **Decreased levels** caused by

- HIV infection

- Sepsis

- Leukemia

- Chemotherapy

**INCREASE IN MONOCYTES MAY BE CAUSED BY;-**

- Tuberculosis

- Chronic inflammatory disease

- Viral infection

**DECREASE IN MONOCYTES MAY BE CAUSED BY:-**

- Blood stream infection

- Bone marrow disorder

- Skin infection

**INCREASE IN EOSINOPHILS MAY B CAUSED BY:-**

- An allergic reaction

- parasitic infection

## ➤ ERYTHROCYTE SEDIMENTATION RATE (ESR)

- ESR is the rate at which red blood cells sediment in a period of one hour. It is common hematology test.

- The ESR is increased in inflammation, pregnancy, anemia, autoimmune disorders (such as rheumatoid arthritis and lupus), infections, some cancers.

- The ESR is decreased in policythemia, sickle cell anemia, leukemia, low plasma protein.

- There are 3 stages in erythrocyte sedimentation:-

- 1) Stage -  1 Rouleaux formation – first 10 min.

- 2) Stage -  2 Sedimentation or settling stage

- 3) Stage - 3 Packing stage

## ➢ **PERIPHERAL EXAMINATION**

- Peripheral smear examined for detailed study of morphology of RBCs and WBCs Abnormal cell seen in tail portion.

- Reporting the peripheral smear;

-	Size
-	Shape
-	Morphology RBCs and WBCs
-	Colour- degree of haemoglobinisation
-	Parasites

**Normocyte:-**

- Normal size RBC.

**Microcyte:-**

- Small size RBC.

- Seen in anaemia eg. Iron deficiency, Thalassaemia.

**Macrocyte:-**

- Large size in RBC

- seen in Aplastic anemia, megaloblastic anaemia, chronic liver disease.

**Tear drop cell:-**

- RBC having one pointed and another blunt end. Seen in anaemia.

**Target cell:-**

- RBC is thin and large concentric circle of rifle target. Seen in severe anaemia,

Spleenectomy, low level of haemoglobin.

**Schistocyte Cell:-**

- RBC cell is irregular shapes seen in thyrotoxicosis etc.

**Acanthocyte cell:-**

- RBC irregular surface of cell seen in abnormal metabolism.

**Ovalocyte cell:-**

- RBC is oval shape. Seen in chronic liver disease, anemias.

**Stomatocyte Cell:-**

- RBC shows like a slit appearance of central biconcave area seen in haemolytic anaemia.

**Elliptocyt:-**

- RBC elliptical in shape seen in hereditary myelosclerosis etc.

**Burr cell:-**

- RBC small or fragmented and few spikes seen in uremia.

## ➢ LUPUS ERYTHEMATOSUS CELL (LE CELL)

- LE cell is a neutrophil or macrophage that has phagocytized the denatured nuclear material of another cell. The denatured material is an absorbed hematoxylin body also called LE body.

- LE cell found in similar connective tissue disorders or some auto immune disease like severe Rheumatoid arthritis.

- ANA (antinuclear antibody) is clearly responsible for the LE cell. Although the auto antibodies cannot penetrate the healthy cells they can attack the nuclei of damaged cells.

- LE factor is an IgG antibody directed against deoxyribonucleic protein. This antibody act on the damaged nucleus producing swelling & homogenisation of nuclear material LE bodies.

**Clinical significance:-**

- Tubular damage
- Viral infection
- Drug toxicity
- Pyelonephritis
- Fever and rash

# MICROBIOLOGY

## ➢ INTRODUCTION OF MICROBIOLOGY

- Micro- organisms or microbes are organisms that are so small (invisible to the naked eye). The study about them is called microbiology.

- Medical microbiology is the study about the microbes and their role in human illness disease causing organisms are called pathogens.

## ➢ STERILIZATION & DISINFECTION

**Sterilization:-**

- A physical or chemical process that completely destroys or removes all microbial life, including spores.

**Disinfection:-**

- It is killing or removing of harmful microorganisms.

**Disinfectant:-**

- Products used to kill microorganisms on inanimate objects or surface. Disinfectants are not necessarily sporicidal, but may be sporostatic, inhibiting germination or outgrowth.

**Methods of sterilization**

2) Physical methods
3) Chemical methods

**Physical methods:-**

- Moist and dry heat
- Radiation

**Chemical methods:-**

- Alcohol, aldehydes, phenol, halogens, heavy metal, dyes.

**Dry heat:-**

- Simplest method is exposing the item to be sterilized to the naked flame

- Hot air oven expose item to 160 c for 1 hr. the oven should be fitted with a thermostat control temperature indicator.

- Used for metals, glassware, ointment, oils, waxes etc.

**Moist heat:-**

Moist heat: - uses hot water, moist heat kill microorganism by denaturing proteins.

**Boiling:-**

- Moist heat may be applied by boiling water or steam. Boiling water is generally used for sterilizing instrument and syringe. These are boiled 10 minutes. In a water bath. This will kill all non- sporing organisms but certain spore forming organisms can resist the temperature of boiling water for 1to 2hr.

**Tyndallisation:-**

- This sterilization is employed by steamer they are exposed to free steaming for 20 min for three successive days. The vegetative bacteria are killed in the first exposure And the spores that germinate by next day are killed in the subsequent days. The success of the process depends on the germination of spores.

**Pasteurization:-**

- It aims to reduce the number of viable pathogens in liquids. It uses heat at temperature sufficient to inactivate harmful organisms in milk. Temperature may be 138 c. or 62c to 35c minutes.

**Autoclaving:-**

- Standard sterilization method in hospitals.

- the autoclave is a tough double walled chamber in which air is replaced by pure saturated steam under pressure.

- The items to be sterilized get completely surrounded by saturated by standard steam which o contact with the surface of material to be sterilized condenses to release its latent heat of condensation which adds to already raised temperature of steam so that eventually all the microorganism in whatever form are killed.

- The usually temperature achieved 121c at pressure 15lbs. At exposure time 15- 20 min. By increasing the temperature. The time sterilizing is further reduced.

**Radiation:-**

- **UV light:** this light limited sterilizing power because of poor penetration into materials generally used in irradiation of air in certain areas e.g. Operating rooms and T.B. laboratories.

- **Non- Ionizing radiation:** Ionizing ray are low energy rays .they used mainly in sterilization of disposable plastic, syringe, gloves, specimen containers and Petri dishes.

- **Ionizing radiation:** Ionizing rays are high energy rays with good penetrative power (E.g. X- rays gamma rays)

**Filtration:** it is method used to remove bacteria from heat labile liquids such as serum, antibiotic solution, sugar solution etc it is achieved by using different types of filter like candle filter, membrane filter, sintered glass filter.

**Chemical:-**
**Alcohols:** - Both ethanol and isopropanol widely used normally at a concentration of about 70%.

- They are bacterial and fungicidal but are not effective against endospores or non- enveloped viruses.

**Silver –sulfadiazine:** - is used in wound dressing .available as topical cream for use on burns.

**Mercuric chloride: -** it's highly bactericidal but is toxic and corrosive and is inactivated by organic matter.

**Formaldehyde: -** Formaldehyde is a high – level disinfectant it is also used anatomy laboratory and preserve anatomic specimens, sterilize surgical instrument.

**Glutaraldehyde: -** Glutaraldehyde is used most commonly as a high – level disinfectant for medical equipment such as endoscope, spirometry tube, Transducer. Glutaraldehyde is noncorrosive to metal and does not damage lenses instruments, rubber or plastic.

**Incineration:-**

- Incineration is useful for disposing of animal carcasses, anatomical and other laboratory waste with or without prior decontamination. That incineration with two combustion chamber are suitable for dealing with infectious materials.

- The temperature in the primary chamber should be at least 800c and that in the secondary chamber at least 1000 c. incineration materials should be transported to the incineration in bags or plastic.

➤ **Infection:-**

- Infection is the invasion lodgement and multiplication of organism in the tissue of host not all infection however results in disease depending on the spread of infection disease.

**CLASSIFICATION OF INFECTIONS**

**1. Primary infection:-**

- Initial infection with organism in host.

**2. Reinfection:-**

- Subsequent infection by same organism in a host (after recovery).

**3. Super infection:-**

- Infection by same organism in a host before recovery.

**4. Secondary infection:-**

- When in a host whose resistance is lowered by pre existing infectious disease.

**5. Focal infection:-**

- It is a condition where due to infection at a localized sites like appendix and tonsil, general effects are produced.

**6. Cross infection:-**

- When a patient is suffering from a disease and new infection is set up from another host or external source.

## ➢ MORPHOLOGY OF BACTERIA

- **Cocci - These** are spherical or oval

- **Monococci** - cocci in singles

- **Staphylococci** - Cocci in grapes like cluster

- **Streptococci** - Cocci in chains

- **Tetrad** - Cocci in group of four

- **Sarcina** - Cocci in group of eight

- **Bacilli** - these are rod – shaped bacteria

- **Vibrio** - coma shaped

- **Actinomycetes:-**

- These are rigid organisms like true bacteria but they resemble fungi in that they exhibit branching and tend to form filaments.

**- Spirochaetes:-**

- These are relatively longer, slender, non- branched microorganism of spiral shape having several coils.

**- Mycoplasmas:-**

- They occur in round or oval bodies and interlacing filament these bacteria lack in rigid cell wall.

**- Aerobes bacteria:-**

- Those bacteria that require oxygen for growth.

**- Obligate anaerobes:-**

- Grow in absence of free oxygen they will die on exposure to even trace amount of oxygen.

**- Obligate aerobe:-**

 - Those bacteria that cannot grow without oxygen for growth

**- Facultative anaerobes:-**

 - They are bacteria that are able to grow in both the presence and absence of oxygen.

**- Microaerophilic:-**

– Requiring little free oxygen or oxygen at a lower partial pressure than that of atmospheric oxygen.

## ➤ VIRUS VS BACTERIA

**VIRUS:-**

- virus are particles that invade your body`s cells

- Viruses contain genetic material (DNA or RNA) and protein coat.

- Viruses take many shapes and are much smaller than bacteria.

- Viruses cause disease such as acute bronchitis, many infections. The body fights against viral infection by producing a fever or inflammation. Antibiotic cannot kill virus.

## BACTERIA:-

- Bacteria is prokaryotic cells.

- **Bacteria** are one of the organisms that take several shapes, rods, spiral they are found everywhere bacteria.

- bacteria cause infections such as invading the body`s cells.

- Bacterial infection need to be treated with an antibiotic, medication that kills bacteria.

# INTRODUCTION TO BACTERIA IDENTIFICATION

- including bacterial identification and pathogen detection is essential for correct disease, diagnosis, treatment of infection.

## ➤ IMPORTANCE OF INDENTIFICATION:-

- Determining the clinical significance of particular pathogen.

- Determining the laboratory testing for detection of antibacterial resistance is warranted.

- Determining the whether infectious organisms are risk for other patients in the hospital, the public and other laboratory workers.

## ➤ IDENTIFICATION METHODS:-

### PHENOTYPIC METHOD:-

- Microscopic morphology and staining characteristics.

- Macroscopic (colony) morphology.

- Environmental requirement for growth.

- Nutritional requirement and metabolic capabilities.

- Resistance or susceptibility to antibacterial agents.

## ➤ SEROLOGICAL METHODS:-

- Immunological methods involve the interaction of a microbial antigen with an antibody (produced by the host immune system).

- Immune testing for agglutination, immune fluorescence, RIA, western blotting, ELISA, precipitation test.

**PRECIPITATION REACTIONS:-**

- Precipitation is the interaction of a soluble Ag with a soluble Ab form an insoluble complex. Ex RPR, VDRL.

**AGGLUTINATION TEST:-**

- Agglutination occurs due to the cross –l linking of particulate antigens by antibody molecules. This agglutination is visible clumping of insoluble particules.

**Immune – fluorescence:-**

- Use fluorescein isothiocyanate labelled immunoglobulin to detect antigen and antibody according to test systems require a fluorescent microscope.

**Enzyme – linked immune- sorbent assay (ELISA):-**

- Use of enzyme labelled immunoglobulin to detect antigens or antibodies.

- Signals are developed by the action of hydrolysing enzyme on chromogenic substrate.

- Optical density measured by micro- plate reader.

## ➢ GENOTYPIC METHODS:-

- The initiation of new molecular technologies in genomics is shifting phynotypic techniques for bacterial classification, identification and characterization.

- PCR, plasmid fingerprinting, nucleic acid probes, RFLP.

# BIOCHEMICAL IDENTIFICATION OF BACTERIA

> **SINGLE ENZYME TEST:-**

- Catalase Test
- Coagulase Test
- Pyrase Test
- Hippurate hydrolysis Test
- Oxidase Test
- Indole Test
- Dnase Test
- ONPG ( B- galactosidase )
- Urease Test

> **CARBOHYDRATE OXIDATION AND FERMENTATION:-**

- Oxidation fermentation Test
- Methyl Red Test
- Voges proskauer Test

## CATALASE TEST:-

- This test is used to differentiate Catalase producing bacteria such as staphylococci from non Catalase producing bacteria such as streptococci.

**Positive test** - rapid and sustained appearance of bubbles of effervescence.

**Negative test -** lack of bubble formation 30 sec later.

## CATALASE POSITIVE BACTERIA:-

- *Staphylococci*

- *Pseudomonas aeroginosa*

- *Aspergillus fumigatus*

- *Candida albicans*

- *Enterobacteriaceae (klebsiella, serratia, shigella, proteus, salmonella, yersinia)*

- *Mycobacterium tuberculosis*

- *Corynebacterium diphtheriae*

- *Cryptococcus and Rhodococcus.*

**Negative Bacteria -** Streptococcus and Enterococcus

## COAGULASE TEST:-

- To determine the ability of the organism to produce Coagulase this clots plasma.

- Coagulase is an enzyme that converts soluble fibrinogen into soluble fibrin.

- **Positive: -** White fibrin clots in plasma (staphylococcus aureus)

- **Negative: -** Smooth suspension (staphylococcus epidermidis)

## COAGULASE TEST POSITIVE BACTERIA:-

- Staphylococcus aureus

- Other animal host like *S. intermedius, S. Delphini, S .lutrae, S. hyicus.*

**Coagulase Negative Bacteria:-**

- *Staphylococcus epidermidis*

- *S. saprophyticus*

- *S. hominis*

**OXIDASE TEST:-**

- This Test is used to help in the identification of the organisms which produce the enzyme Oxidase.

- **Positive Test: -** blue / dark purple / black colour (Pseudomonas aeruginosa)

- **Negative Test: -** No colour development (*E.COLI*)

**OXIDASE TEST POSITIVE BACTERIA:-**

- *Pseudomonas aeruginosa*

- *Neisseria*

- *Alcaligens*

- *Aeromonas*

- *Campylobacter*

- *Vibrio cholerae*

- *Brucella*

- *Pasteurella*

- *Helicobacter pylori*

**OXIDASE NEGATIVE BACTERIA:-**

- *Enterobacteriaceae (ex. E.coli)*

**PYRASE (PYR) TEST:-**

- To determine the ability of the organism to hydrolyze the substrate L-pyrrolidonyl- beta- napthylamide

- To differentiate the ***Enterococcus*** species from the ***Nonenterococcus*** species.

- **Positive Test: -** Pink to cheery red colour (after addition of colour developer)

- **Negative Test: -** No colour change.

## PYRASE TEST POSITIVE BACTERIA:-

- *Enterococcus faecalies*

- *Enterococcus faecium*

- *Enterococcus avium*

## PYRASE TEST NEGATIVE BACTERIA:-

- *Streptococcus agalactiae*

- *S. bovis*

- *S. milleri*

## HIPPURATE HYDROLYSIS TEST:-

- To determine the ability of the organism to produce hippuricase which hydrolyzes the substrate Hippurate.

- Useful in the identification of ***streptococcus agalactiae*** and ***comphylibacter jejuni*** and ***listeria monocytogenes.***

- This test also differentiation of beta – hemolytic streptococcus agalactiae from other beta hemolytic streptococci

- **Positive Test: -** deep purple colour (streptococcus *agalactiae)*

- **negative Test: -** slightly yellow pink or colourless (*enterococcus*)

## HIPPURATE HYDROLYSIS TEST POSITIVE BACTERIA:-

- *Campylobacter jejuni*

- *Listeria monocytogenes*

- *Streptococcus agalactiae*

**HIPPURATE HYDROLYSIS TEST NEGATIVE BACTERIA:-**

- *Streptococcus pyogenes*

- *Campylobacter coli*

**INDOLE TEST:-**

- To distinguish Enterobacteriaceae based on the ability to produce Indole from tryptophan.

- To identify lactose fermenting member of *Enterobacteriaceae, E.coli Klebsiella pneumonia.*

**Positive test:** - Red ring at the interface of reagent

**Negative test:** - No colour development

**INDOLE TEST POSITIVE BACTERIA:-**

- *E.coli*

- *Proteus vulgaris*

- *Vibrio cholarae*

- *Enterococcus faecalis*

- *Aeromonas hydrophilia*

- *Bacillus alvei*

**INDOLE TEST NEGATIVE BACTERIA:-**

- *Klebsiella aerogenes*

- *K. pneumonia*

- *Proteus mirabilis*

- *Salmonella typhi*

- *Salmonella Para typhi A*

- *Enterobacter sp*

- *Serrattia marcescens*

## DNA HYDROLYSIS TEST (DNase):-

- To detect Dnase Activity in species of aerobic bacteria.

- To differentiate non fermenting gram- negative bacteria as well as staphylococcus aureus which produce the enzyme deoxiribonuclease from other staphylococci which do not produce DNase.

- **Positive Test: -** Rose pink and clear zone

- **Negative Test: -** No change and no clearing

### DNase test positive bacteria:-

- *Staphylococcus aureus*

- *Streptococcus pyogenes*

- *Moraxella catarrhalis*

- *Serratia species*

- *Aeromonas*

- *Vibro*

### DNase TEST NEGATIVE BACTERIA:-

- *Staphylococcus epidermidis*

- *Klebsiella*

- *Enterobacter*

- *E.coli*

### ONPG (B- GALACTOSIDASE TEST):-

- To determine the presence of late or slow fermenting strains.

- To detect the late lactose fermenting strains of Escherichia coli

**Positive Test: -** yellow colour within 20 min to 24 hr

**Negative Test: -** No colour change or colourless after 24 hr

## ONPG TEST POSITIVE BACTERIA:-

- *E.coli*

- *Klebsiella spp*

- *Enterobacter Spp*

- *Cirtobacter spp*

## ONPG TETS NEGATIVE BACTERIA:-

- *Salmonella spp.*

- *Shigella spp.*

- *Proteus spp.*

- *Morganella spp.*

**Urease Test:-**

- To determine the ability of an organism to produce the enzyme, Urease which hydrolyzes urea.

- To identify the rapid Urease produce proteus and Morganella

- **Positive Test: -** Red colour in the medium (broth)

- **Negative Test: -** No colour change

## UREASE TEST POSITIVE BACTERIA:-

- *Proteus spp.*

- *Klebsiella spp.*

- *Cryptococcus spp.*

- *Helicobacter pylori.*

## UREASE TEST NEGATIVE BACTERIA:-

- *E.coli*

- *Shigella*

- *Salmonella typhi*

- *V. cholera*

- *Enterobacter sp.*

## OXIDATION –FERMENTATION ( O- F) TEST :-

- This test is used to differentiate the organisms that oxidize carbohydrate (aerobic utilization) from those organisms that ferment carbohydrates (anaerobic utilization)

- Differentiation of Pseudomonas aeruginosa (carbohydrate oxidation), Enterobacteriaceae (carbohydrate fermentation).

**Test positive :- 1)** yellow green - oxidative organisms (aerobic)

 2) Yellow to yellow fermentative – fermentative (anaerobic)

**Negative Test: -** No utilization carbohydrate.

## O- F TEST POSITIVE BACTERIA:-

- *Pseudomonas aeruginosa* (Oxidative positive)

- *Escherichia coli* (fermentative positive)

## TRIPLE SUGAR IRON AGAR:-

- As an initial step in the identification of Enterobacteriaceae.

- The action of many species of microorganisms on a carbohydrate substrate results in the acidification of the medium with or without gas formation.

**Yellow / Yellow, Acid / Acid. (Gas – positive, H2s – Negative)**

- Glucose fermented - *Escherichia coli*

- Lactose or sucrose fermented - *Klebsiella spp.*

- Lactose or sucrose fermented - *Enterobacter sp*

**Yellow / Yellow, Acid /Acid (Gas – Positive, H2s – Positive)**

- Glucose and sucrose fermented - *Proteus vulgaris*

**Red / Yellow, Alkaline / Acid (Gas – Negative, H2s – Negative)**

- Glucose fermented - Shigella sp

- Lactose or sucrose not fermented - *Proteus morganii, proteus rettgeri*

**Red / Yellow, Alkaline / Acid (Gas – Negative, H2s – Positive)**

- Glucose fermented - *Salmonella typhi*

- Lactose or sucrose not fermented - *Salmonella typhi*

**Red / Yellow, Alkaline / Acid (Gas – Positive, H2s – Positive)**

- Glucose Fermented - *Other Salmonella sp*

- Lactose or Sucrose not fermented - *Proteus mirabilis*

**Red / Yellow, Alkaline / Acid (Gas – Positive, H2s – Negative)**

- Glucose fermented - Providencia alcalifaciens

- Lactose or Sucrose not Fermented - Providencia alcalifaciens

**Red / Red, Alkaline / Alkaline (Gas – Negative, H2s – Negative)**

- None of the sugar fermented - Do not belong to Enterobacteriaceae

## METHYL RED TEST:-

- Some bacteria have the ability to utilize glucose and convert it to a stable acid like lactic acid, acetic acid, or formic acid as the end product.

- This Test is performed to differentiate Enterobacteria

**Test positive** – distinct red colour at surface of the medium

**Test Negative** – Yellow colour at the surface of the medium

## METHYL RED TEST POSITIVE BACTERIA:-

- *E.coli*

- *K.pneumoniae*

- *P. vulgaris*

- *Salmonella Typhi*

- *Shigella sp*

## METHYL RED TEST NEGATIVE BACTERIA:-

- *K. aerogenes*

- *P.mirabilis*

- *V.cholerae*

- *P.aeruginosa*

## VOGES PROSKAUER TEST:-

- This test is used to assist in the differentiation of Enterobacteria.

- The presence of oxygen and 40% potassium hydroxide, acetone is converted to the diacetyl form, which result in a Red colour in the presence of alpha –napthol.

**Test positive:** - pink red colour at surface of the medium

**Test Negative:** - Yellow colour at surface of the medium

**VP TEST POSITIVE BACTERIA:-**

- *Enterobacter*

- *Klebsiella*

- *V.cholerae*

- *Serratia marcescens*

**VP TEST NEGATIVE BACTERIA:-**

- *E.coli*

- *K.pneumoniae*

- *Salmonella typhi*

- *Shigella sp*

- *Yersinia*

## CITRATE UTILIZATION TEST:-

- Citrate test the ability of organisms to utilize citrate as a carbon source.

- This test is performed in the identification of the lactose fermenting Enterobacteria.

**Positive Test: -** growth with an intense blue colour on the slant

**Negative Test: -** absence of growth and no colour change.

## CITRATE UTILIZATION TEST POSITIVE BACTERIA:-

- *K.aerogenes*

- *K.pneumoniae*

- *P.mirabilis*

- *Enterobacter spp*

- *Serratia marcescens*

## CITRATE UTILIZATION TEST NEGATIVE BACTERIA:-

- *E.coli*

- *Salmonella typhi*

- *Shigella*

- *Salmonella paratyphi A*

# MEDIA

> **SELECTIVE MEDIA:-**

- A growth medium or culture medium is a solid liquid or semi – solid designed to support the growth of microorganism or cells.

> **TRANSPORT MEDIA:-**

- Transport media are special media preserve a specimen and minimize bacterial over growth from the time of collection to the time it is received at the laboratory to be processed.

> **ENRICHED MEDIA :-**

- Enriched media contain the nutrients required to support the growth of a wide variety of organism. They are commonly used to harvest as many types of microbes as present in the specimen.

> **DIFFERENTIAL MEDIA:-**

- A growth medium or culture medium is a solid, liquid or semi – solid designed to support the growth of microorganism or cells.

> **DIFFERENT TYPES OF CULTURE MEDIA:-**

**MEDIA MAIN USE**

- Alkaline peptone water Enrichment media vibrio cholera

- Alkaline salt Transport media

- Thio sulphate citrate bile salt sucrose agar (TCBS) Selective media

- Blood agar Indicator media

- Castaneda media Isolation of brucella

- Crystal violate blood agar Selective media for streptococcus pyogenes

- Cysteine lactose electrolyte deficient media (CLED) Culturing urine samples

- Yolk agar Detection of lipase activity of clostridium species.

- Blood Agar Beta- hemolytic streptococcus

- Charcoal blood agar Isolation of bordetella pertussis

- Campylobacter thioglycollate broth Selective media of campylobacter species

- Castaneda medium isolation of brucella

- Levinthal`s agar Haemophilus Influenza

- Tinsdale medium Isolation of Corynebacterium from throat swabs

- Lowenstein Jensen medium (LJ) Isolation of mycobacterium

- MacConkey agar differential media for enterobacteriaceae

- Wilson and Blair's brilliant green bismuth sulphate (BBSA) Differential and media for isolation of salmonella & shigella stool specimens

- Muller – Hinton agar Performing antimicrobial susceptibility for bacteria

- Nutrient agar supports the growth of all non fastidious organisms

- Non – nutrient agar Cultivation of parasites

- Pike`s media Preservation of S.pyogens, Pneumococci, hemophilus

- Robertson cooked meat broth (RCMB) Growth of anaerobes

- Thayer – martin medium Neisseria gonorrhoea

- Triple sugar iron agar (TSI) medium Differential of various Members of Enterobacteriaceae

- Wilkins – chalgren agar Performing antimicrobial susceptibility of anaerobic bacteria

# PARASITE

## ➢ PARASITE INTRODUCTION:-

- The study of parasites that cause disease in man is called as medical parasitology.

- Clinical parasitology deals with those pathogenic organisms which are bigger in size than bacteria and fungi.

- The host in which the sexual phase is seen is called the definitive host.

- parasitic infection in man primarily involve in the intestine but can also included urogenital tract, muscle, and other organs.

- Specimen which are tested for the parasites are –

- Stool
- Urine
- Blood
- Sputum
- Urogenital swab

## ➢ PARASITIC INFECTION:-

- Parasitic are organisms that live off other organisms or host to survive, some parasite don`t found affect their hosts. Other grow, reproduces, invade organ system that makes their hosts sick resulting in a parasitic infection.

- The symptoms of parasitic infection very depending on the organism.

- parasitic infection can be caused by three types of organism.

1) Protozoa
2) Helminths
3) Ectoparasites

- Protozoa are single – celled organism that can live and multiply inside your body.

- Helminths are multi- celled organism that can live in or outside of your body.

- Ectoparasites are multi- celled organism that live on or feed off your skin. They include some insects and such as mosquitos, mites.

➢ **PROTOZOA :-**

➢ <u>**NAME**</u>

- Entamoeba histolytica

<u>**BODY PARTS AFFECT:-**</u>

- Intestine -

<u>**DIAGNOSTIC SPECIMEN:-**</u>

- stool

➢ <u>**NAME**</u>

- Leishmania spp.

<u>**BODY PARTS AFFECT**</u>

- Visceral or cutaneous

<u>**DIAGNOSTIC SPECIMEN:-**</u>

- Visual identification

➢ <u>**NAME**</u>

- Malaria

<u>**BODY PARTS AFFECT**</u>

- Red blood cell

<u>**DIAGNOSTIC SPECIMEN:-**</u>

- Blood smear

➢ **<u>NAME</u>**

- Toxoplasma gondii

**<u>BODY PARTS AFFECT</u>**

- Eyes, brain, heart, liver

**<u>DIAGNOSTIC SPECIMEN:-</u>**

- Blood or PCR

➢ **<u>NAME</u>**

- Giardia lambila

**<u>BODY PARTS AFFECT</u>**

- small intestine

**<u>DIAGNOSTIC SPECIMEN:-</u>**

- stool

➢ **<u>NAME</u>**

- Trichomonas vaginalis

**<u>BODY PARTS AFFECT</u>**

- urogenital tract (female)

**<u>DIAGNOSTIC SPECIMEN:-</u>**

- Genital swab

➢ **<u>NAME</u>**

- Babesia. Bovis

**<u>BODY PARTS AFFECT</u>**

- red blood cell

**<u>DIAGNOSTIC SPECIMEN:-</u>**

- Blood smear

**Protozoa life cycle:-**

- Microbe enters the body from the source water, soli, food, from animal or other humans.

- Microbe penetrating into the body of the new owner, begins to multiply there creating a lot of new parasites.

- Microbe lay eggs in the body.

- Parasites can cause the following symptoms:-

- Nausea
- Vomiting
- Diarrhoea
- Other gastrointestinal problems

> **HELMINTHS:-**

- Three types of Helminths

1) Nematod (Round worms)
2) Trematode (Flukes)
3) Cestoda (Tape worm)

**Nematod:-**

| Name | Affect body parts | Diagnostic specimen |
|---|---|---|
| - **Necator americanus** | Lungs, Small intestine, | Stool |
| - **Ascaris lumbricoides** | Intestine, liver, Stool, lungs, pancreas, | Stool |
| - **Enterobius vermicularis** | Intestine, Anus, | Stool |

**Trematoda:-**

| Name | Affect body parts | Diagnostic specimen |
|---|---|---|
| - **Fasciola hepatica** | Liver, Stool, | Blood |
| - **Fasciolopsis buski** | Intestine, | Stool |
| - **Schistosoma** | Blood flukes, | Stool or urine |

**Cestoda:-**

| Name | Affect body parts | Diagnostic specimen |
|---|---|---|
| - **Necator americanus** | Lungs, Small intestine, | Stool |
| - **Ascaris lumbricoides** | Intestine, Anus, | Stool |
| - **Enterobius vermicularis** | Intestine, Anus, | Stool |
| - **Toxocara canis** | Liver, Brain, Eyes Blood, | Ocular examination |
| - **Trichuris trichiura** | Large intestine, Anus, | Stool |

**Helminths life cycle:-**

- Three main life cycle stages

1) Eggs
2) Larvae
3) Adults


- Infective stages: - Egg or larva

- Definitive Host: - Harbours adult stage

- Intermediate Host: - May be more than one

**Symptoms:-**

- Poor appetite
- Intermittent abdominal pain
- Diarrhoea
- Colonic ulceration
- Iron deficiency anaemia

**ECTOPARASITES LIFE CYCLE :-**

**Name Affected body parts Diagnostic body parts**

- Pediculus human's Hair follicles Visual identification

- Pthirus pubis Pubic area, eyelashes Visual identification

- Cimex lectularius Skin Visual identification

**Ectoparasites life cycle :-**

- This life cycle which takes about 3 to 4 weeks, occur on the host.

- Lice can live for only about a week in the absence of the host.

- Louse eggs, cemented to animal hair, hatch as nymphs, which are small, immature adults.

- The nymph moults three times before becoming adults.

**Symptoms:-**

- Itching and scratching
- Loss of hair in various areas or all over the body.
- Various types of skin eruption, some of which are crusty and may ooze pus or even bleed.
- Scratching of ears.

# SEROLOGY TEST

## C- REACTIVE PROTEIN (CRP):-

- CRP is a substance produced by the liver in response to inflammation .high level of CRP in the blood is a marker of inflammation.

- CRP levels can be elevated in any inflammatory condition.

CRP reading of greater than 10 mg/L is especially high and may indicate:-

- Bone infection or osteomyelitis
- Autoimmune arthritis ( RA )
- Tuberculosis
- Lupus
- Cancer, especially lymphoma
- Pneumonia or other significant infection

- CRP found during viral infection compared to bacterial infections.

- CRP is more sensitive and accurate reflection of the acute phase response than the ESR, ESR may be normal while CRP is elevated.

## Anti – streptolysin O (ASO):-

- ASO is the antibody made against streptolysin O, an immunogenic, oxygen – labile streptococcal hemolytic exotoxin produced by most strain of streptococcus bacteria .

- the "O" in the name stands for oxygen- labile; the main function of streptolysin –O is to cause hemolysis (the breaking open of red blood cells) in particular beta – hemolysis.

- Increased levels of also titre in the blood could cause damage to the heart and joints.

- When the body is infected with streptococci it produce antibodies against the various antigens that the streptococci produce.

- It is done by serological methods like latex agglutination or slide agglutination .ELISA may be performed to detect the exact titre value.

- ASO is a measure of the blood plasma levels of antistreptolysin O antibodies used in test for the diagnose of a streptococcal infection or indicate a past exposure to streptococci.

**Syphilis (VDRL):-**

- Syphilis is a sexually transmitted disease (STD) caused by an infection with bacteria known as Treponema pallidum.

- STD can be spread by any type of sexual contact and also infected mother to the fetus during pregnancy or to the baby at the time of birth it can cause long- term damage to different organs if not properly treated.

- Treponema palladium are referred to as spirochetes due to their spiral shape. The organisms penetrate into the lining of the mouth or genital area.

- There are two types of test used to diagnoses syphilis. The blood test used to syphilis are called the venereal disease research laboratory (VDRL) these test detect the body's response to the Infection.

- STD can present in of four different stages primary, secondary, latent, and tertiary.

**HUMAN IMMUNODEFICIENCY VIRUS (HIV):-**

- HIV is found throughout all the tissues of the body but is transmitted via the body fluids of an infected person (semen, vaginal fluids, blood, and breast milk.)

- HIV is the virus which attacks the T – cells in the immune system .HIV is different in structure from other retroviruses.

- It is roughly spherical with a diameter of about 120nm around 60 times smaller than a red blood cell.

- This is in turn surrounded by the viral envelope that is composed of the lipid bilayer taken from the membrane of a human host cell when the newly formed virus particle buds from the cells.

- HIV transmitted by sexual transmission, perinatal transmission, blood transmission.

**SYMPTOMS OF HIV INFECTION:-**

- Fever, chills, joint pain, muscle aches, sore throat, sweats particularly night, tiredness, weakness, weight loss, dry cough, diarrhoea, shortness of breath .

**ACQUIRED IMMUNODEFICIENCY SYNDROME (AIDS):-**

- A disease of the immune system due to infection with HIV.

- AIDS is an advanced stage of infection with the HIV.

- AIDS is the final stage of HIV infection.

- The most common opportunistic infection In AIDS patient include the following

**Bacterial infection** - caused by mycobacterium tuberculosis, Salmonella species, Nocardia asteroides.

- **Fungal infection** – caused by Candida albicans, Cryptococcus neoformans.

- **Protozonal infection** – Toxoplasma gondii, isospora belli.

- **Viral infection** - Herpes simplex virus, cytomegalovirus, hepatitis B virus.

- AIDS patient and it is characterized by poor memory, apathy, inability to concentrate, and behavioral changes.

**RHEMATOID ARTHRITIS (RA):-**

- Rheumatoid arthritis is an autoimmune disease that causes inflammation of your joints.

- RA is a chronic condition that cause a variety of symptoms including –

- Joint pain
- Joint stiffness
- Limited mobility
- Swelling
- Fatigue
- Feeling of discomfort or not being well

- Inflammation and joint pain can attack different parts of your body such as the joints in your hands and feet, in some cases RA causes inflammation in organs like your lungs or eyes.

- RA positive means that blood tests show the presence of anti- cylic citrullinated peptides (Anti CCPs), also called Anti- citrullinated protein antibodies (ACPAs).

- Anti CCPs are antibodies produced against proteins in the body undergoing a molecular change in structure called citrullination . They are present in approximately 60 to 80 % of people diagnosed with RA.

## ➢ **RAPID PLASMA REAGIN (RPR):-**

- A RPR test is a blood test used to syphilis. It works by detecting the nonspecific antibodies that your body produce to fight the infection.

- Syphilis is a sexually transmitted infection caused by the spirochete bacterium, Treponema pallidum.

- Non - reactive: - smooth suspension No clumping.

- Reactive: - Any degree of clumping

- RPR test is a macroscopic, nontreponemal flocculation card test used to screen for syphilis.

## ➢ MALARIA:-

- Malaria is a typically transmitted through the bite of an infected anopheles.

- Five types of plasmodium parasites can infect humans.

- Malaria symptoms can be classified in to two categories

1) Uncomplicated
2) Severe malaria.

### Uncomplicated

- This is diagnosed when symptoms are present but there are no signs to indicate severe infection.

- Symptoms of uncomplicated malaria typically last 6 to 10 hr and recur every second day.

- In uncomplicated malaria, symptoms progress as follows,

- Fever
- Headaches and vomiting
- Cold, hot, sweating
- Tiredness

### Severe malaria:-

- In severe malaria signs of vital organ dysfunction

- Fever and chills
- Impaired consciousness
- Deep breathing
- Clinical jaundice

### Dengue Fever:-

- Dengue fever is mosquito's tropical disease caused by the dengue virus.

- Dengue is spread by several species of mosquito. Dengue is caused by a RNA virus. This virus is a member of the viral family flaviviridae. Genome contain 11000 nucleotide bases.

- Transmitted by aedes mosquito`s. This mosquito is the obligate intermediate host for some viruses.

- Biting around the ankles and knees. Only female mosquito will bite and mostly in the day time.

- Aedes albopictus are generally associated with the spread of dengue fever. This mosquito black and white stripes on its body and legs, lays its eggs in clean, stagnant water.

**Symptoms of Dengue fever:-**

- High fever, headache
- Vomiting
- Muscle and joint pains
- Skin rash

**Dengue hemorrhagic fever (DHF) :-**

- Bleeding from nose, mouth
- Low levels of platelets
- Blood plasma leakage

**Dengue shock syndrome (DSS)**

- The most severe form of the disease
- Severe abdominal pain
- Heavy bleeding
- A sudden drop in blood pressure (Shock) death.

**Diagnosis for dengue :-**

- Detection of antibodies against virus
- Complete blood count
- Liver function test

**Chikungunya:-**

- Chikungunya is an infection caused by the Chikungunya virus. These typically occur 2 or 12 days after exposure.

- The virus is spread between people by two types of mosquitos Aedes albopictus and aedes aegypti they mainly bite during the day.

- The virus may circulated within a number of animals including birds.

- Diagnosis is by either testing the blood for the virus RNA or antibodies to the virus.

- Chikungunya virus can cause brain inflammation and death in some people.

**Symptoms:-**

- Sudden onset with high fever
- Joint pain and rash
- Headache
- Fatigue
- Digestive complaints
- Conjunctivitis
- Nausea, vomiting,diarrhoea

**Typhoid:-**

- Typhoid fever is a type of enteric fever along with paratyphoid fever. The cause is the bacterium salmonella typhi, also known as salmonella enteric fever.

- The bacterium lives in the intestine and blood stream of human.

- Typhoid is spread by eating or drinking food or water contaminated with feces of an infected person.

- S.typhi enters through the mouth and spends 1 to 3 week in the intestine after this, It makes its way through the intestinal wall and into the blood stream. it spread into other tissue and organs.

- Typhoid is diagnose by detecting the presence of S.typhi via blood, stool and urine.

**Symptoms:-**

- High fever and rash
- Weakness
- Abdominal pain
- Constipation
- Headaches
- Vomiting

**TORCH TEST:-**

- A mother can pass infections to a fetus during pregnancy or delivery. Early detection and treatment of these infections is crucial or preventing complication in the newborn.

- This test may also used to detect disease in infants.

- TORCH is five infections covered in the screening:

 1) Toxoplasmosis

2) Other disease, including HIV, syphilis and measles

3) Rubella

4) Cytomegalo virus

5) Herpes simplex.

- These particular diseases can cross the placenta and cause birth defect in the born.

- The test screen for antibodies to infectious disease. Antibodies are proteins that recognize and destroy harmful substances, such as viruses and bacteria. The presence of certain antibodies usually indicates a current or recent infection.

**HERPES VIRUS:-**

- Herpes virus large family of DNA viruses that cause disease in animal including humans.

- The herpes viruses that commnaly infect human include –

1) **Herpes simplex virus - 1 (HSV- 1):-** Primary Target cell mucoepithelial cell, oral or genital herpes, and spread of sexually transmitted infection.
2) **Herpes simplex virus - 2 ( HSV – 2 ) :-** Primary Target cell mucoepithelial cell, oral or genital as well as other herpes simplex infection and close contact oral or sexually transmitted disease .
3) **Varicella – zoster virus (VZV):-** Primary Target cell mucoepithelial cell, chickenpox and shingles respiratory and close contact.
4) **Epstein – Barr virus (EBV):-** primary Target cell B cell and epithelial cells, infectious CNS lymphoma in AIDS patients, lymphoproliferative syndrome.
5) **Cytomegalo virus (CMV):-** Primary Target cell monocytes and epithelial cells, infectious mononucleosis like syndrome, retinitis, saliva, urine, blood, Breast milk.
6) **Roseolo virus, herpes lymphotropic virus: -** Target cell T Cells, drug – induced hypersensitivity syndrome, hepatitis infection.
7) **Kaposi`s sarcoma associated herpes viruses (KSHV):-** Target cell Lymphocyte and other cells, close contact sexual.

**RUBELLA VIRUS:-**

- Rubella also known as German measles or three day measles is an infection caused by the Rubella virus.

- Is usually starts on the face and spreads to the body the rash is sometimes is itchy, swollen lymph nodes are common and may last a few weeks, a fever, sore throat and fatigue may also occur.

- Rubella is usually spread through the air via cough of the people are infected.

- Rubella is preventable with the rubella vaccine with a single dose being more than 95% effective often it is given in combination with the measles vaccine and mumps vaccine known is MMR vaccine.

- Rubella infection are prevented by the active immunisation programs using live attenuated virus vaccine.

# STAINING


## ➢ GRAM STAINING:-

- This staining technique helps to determine.

1) Gross morphology of the bacteria.
2) Differentiation of bacteria into the two groups (Gram negative, Gram positive).

- This differentiation is helpful In determining the subsequent biochemical tests and media for their culture in the laboratory.

- the alcohol treatment decolorizes gram negative bacteria while gram positive bacteria retain the colour purple.

## ➢ ACID – FAST STAINING :-

- The organisms such as mycobacterium tuberculosis and mycobacterium leprae are extremely difficult to stain by ordinary methods because of the lipid containing cell wall.

- They bind carbol- fuchsin tightly and resist destaining with strong decolorizing agents such as alcohol and strong acid.

- Acid fast negative bacteria readily lose the stain when treated with acid - alcohol solution.

- Heat is applied in the ziehl – Nielsen hot stain method for the detection of M.tuberculosis and cold stain method is used for the detection of M.leprae.

## ALBERT STAINING :-

- Corynebacterium is the genus of gram positive, non acid fast, non motile bacilli, Non sporing. The most important member of the genus is Corynebacterium the causative agent of diphtheria.

- In sputum slide Alberts staining is use.

- The bacterial cell of Corynebacterium diphtheria cytoplasm is neutral.

- Albert stain have two dyes "Toluidine blue O ""malachite green "both of which are basic dyes.

## HAEMATOXYLIN AND EOSIN STAINING (H&E):-

- H & E staining is used histology to examine thin section of tissue.

- Haematoxylin stains cell nuclei blue while eosin stains cytoplasm, connective tissue and other extracellular substance pink and red.

- Hematoxylin stains the cell nucleus and other acidic structures blue. In contrast, eosin stains the cytoplasm and collagen pink.

### ➢ PAPANICOLAOU STAIN (PAP):-

- PAP stain is a multichromatic staining cytological technique developed by George papanikolaou the father of cytopathology.

- Pap staining is used to differentiate cells in smear preparation of various bodily secretions. The specimen can be gynaecological smears.

- PAP staining is very reliable technique. As such it is used for cervical cancer screening in gynecology. The entire procedure is known as Pap smear.

### ➢ ROMANOWSKY STAINS:-

- Romanowsky stains are neutral stains composed of a mixture of oxidized methylene blue dyes and eosin.

- Blood films, bone marrow examination, cytology.

- The Romanowsky stains is that they impart a reddish purple colour to the chromatin of malaria and other parasites.

### ➢ SUDAN BLACK B :-

- Sudan black B is a dye that is insoluble in water but dissolves in fat therefore this dye will accumulate in fat globules within cells.

- It is slightly basic dye and will combine with acidic groups in compound lipids, thus staining phospholipids also.

- Fat is blue / black

- Nuclei Red.

## ➢ PERIODIC ACID – SCHIFF ( PAS ) :-

- PAS is a staining method used to detect polysaccharides such as glycogen and mucosubstance such as glycoproteins, glycolipids and mucins in tissue.

- PAS staining is mainly used for staining structure containing a high proportion of carbohydrate macromolecules.

- PAS staining is also used for staining cellulose.

## ➢ CAPSULE STAINING:-

- The main purpose of capsule stain is to distinguish capsular material from the bacterial cell. A capsule is a gelatinous outer layer secreted by bacterial cell and that surrounds and adheres to the cell wall.

- Most capsules are composed of polysaccharides but some are composed of polypeptides.

- The capsule stain employs an acidic stain and basic stain to detect capsule production.

- Negative staining methods contrast a translucent, darker colored, background with stained cells but an unstained capsule. The background formed with India ink or nigrosin or Congo red.

- Positive capsule stain requires a mordent that precipitates the capsule. By counterstaining with dyes like crystal violet or methylene blue, bacterial cell wall takes up the dye.

- Positive capsule ex, bacillus, anthracis, klebsiella pneumonia, neisseriae meningitis.

- Negative capsule ex, Neisseria gonorrhoea.

> ## SPIROCHETES STAINING (FONTANA`S METHOD):-

- Spirochete are gram Negative, flexible, spiral shaped organisms who have distinct morphology and mechanism of locomotion.

- Delicate nature of spirochetes heat fixation is avoided as it destroys the shape of organisms .chemical like formalin and glacial acetic acid are used for fixation.

- Mordant containing tannic acid increase the affinity of stain towards the cell. Finally when the stain containing ammoniacal silver nitrate is heat up, silver oxide is formed which precipitates on the organism thereby the apparent diameter is adequately increase and organism are visible.

- Spirochete are stained brownish black in colour against brown background.

> ## PROBLEMS OF STAINING:-

**- Excessively Blue stain**:

**Cause**: too thick films, prolonged staining, inadequate, washing too high alkalinity

**Appearance**: Erythrocytes blue green nuclear chromatin deep blue to black granules of neutrophil deeply stained and appear large and prominent.

**Correction:** Preparing films with ideal thickness reducing staining time using less stain and more diluents prolonging washing adjust pH of buffer.

**- Excessively pink stain:**

**Cause:** insufficient staining prolonged washing too high acidity of the stain or buffer.

**Appearance:** Erythrocytes bright red or orange nuclear chromatin pale blue granules of Eosinophils brilliant red.

**Correction:** Prolonged staining time reducing, washing, preparing, a new batch stain.

**Precipitate on the film:-**

- **Cause:** unclean slides, drying, during the period of staining inadequate washing of slide at the end of the staining period.

- **Correction:** use clean slides cover the smear with generous amount of the stain wash the slide until thinner parts of the film are pinkish.

# HISTOLOGY

## ➢ INTRODUCTION OF HISTOLOGY:-

- Histology technique deals with the preparation of tissue for microscopic examination.

- Make them hard so that very thin section (4 to 5 micron) can be made.

- Good staining should be possible.

- After staining the section should represent the anatomy of the tissue as close to as possible to their structure in life.

- This is achieved by passing the total as selected part of the tissue through a series of process.

### Biopsy:-

The removal of a sample of tissue for examination under a microscope to check for cancer cells or other abnormalities.

### Autopsy:-

- A post mortem examination to discover the cause of death or the extent of disease.

## ➢ HISTORY FOLLOWED IN HISTOLOGY:-

### - Identification:-

Tissue specimen received In the laboratory have a request form that lists the patient information.

### - Labelling of the specimen:-

The specimen is decessioned by giving them a number that will identify each specimen for each patient.

**Grossing:-**

- The specimen is then cut into representative is put in small plastic or still cassette to hold the tissue then processor.

> **GROSS EXAMINATION OF TISSUE:-**

- The term "Grossing" means inspecting the specimens describing and measuring the tissue.

- First the patient information on the requisition and on the specimen container must match in entirely. This includes at least three patient identifiers as well as the specimen site, requisitions typically identify the surgical procedure then the cassette number or bar code must match the specimen as well as the requisition.

- The grossing must be well ventilated to prevent inhalation of formaldehyde fumes, personal protective equipment should include disposable gloves and lab coat as well as protective eye wear. Blades and sharps used during grossing must be disposed of in approved biohazardous waste containers.

- One specimen container should be opened at one time during grossing to prevent mixups.

- The number of pieces in each container should be noted.

- The colour description consistency, appearance and any apparent abnormalities.

- Tissue should be sectioned according to accepted protocols for the laboratory generally the section should be approximately 3-4 mm thick/ wide.

- Microscopic examination of tissue in order to study the manifestation or disease.

> ➤ **VARIOUS TYPES OF MICROTOMES:-**

**Rotary microtome:-**

- USE: steel glass or diamond blades depending upon the specimen being sliced and the desired thickness of the section being cut.

**Rocking microtome:-**

- USE: the easiest to use microtome capable of producing section down to 5 microns of wax.

**Base- sledge microtome:-**

USE: used in botanical microtome technique where hard materials like bone. These microtomes have heavier blades and cannot cut thin as a regular microtome.

**Sliding microtome:-**

USE: sliding microtome holds the block and the knife is moved along the horizontal plane .as the knife is returned to the starting position, it complete each section cycle.

The block tube toward the knife at a predetermined thickness.

**Freezing microtome:-**

USE: This microtome facilitates applications in both the histology and research labs.

Freezing microtome are used for sectioning fresh frozen tissues without embedding procedure.

**Cryostat microtome:-**

USE: It is use for fast pathological examination. Tissue containing large amount of water section best at warmer temperature.

**Vibrating microtome:-**

USE: The vibrating microtome operates by cutting using a vibrating blade. This microtome is usually used for difficult biological samples.

**Saw microtome:-**

USE: saw microtome is especially for hard materials such as teeth and bones.

**Ultra- microtome:-**

USE: used for very thin section. The typically thickness of tissue cut is between 20 to 100 nm. Diamond or glass knife use.

# HISTOLOGY TECHNIQUE

1) Fixation
2) Dehydration
3) Cleaning
4) Embedding
5) Cutting
6) Staining

**FIXATION:-**

- To prevent autolysis and bacterial attack.

- To fix the tissue so they will not change their volume and shape during processing.

- To prepare tissue and leave it in condition which allows clear staining of section.

- To leave tissue as close as their living state as possible and no small molecules should be lost.

**Classification of fixatives:-**

1) Simple fixative: - Aldehydes, formaldehyde, glutaraldehyde.
2) Oxidizing agent :- Potassium permanganate, Potassium dichromate
3) Protein denaturing agent or coagulant :- Acetic acid,Methyl alcohol,Ethyl alcohol
4) Other: - Mercuric chloride, picric acid, non- aldehydes containing fixative.

**Following factors are important:**

1) Solid organ :-

- cut slice as necessary as but not thicker than 5mm.

2) Hollow organ :-

- either open or fill with fixative or pack lightly with wool soaked in fixative.

3) Large specimen :-

- It require dissection, inject fixative along the vessels or bronchi as in case of lung so that reaches all parts of the organs.

- The speed of fixation of most fixative is almost 1mm/hr.

## DEHYDRATION:-

- To remove fixative and water from the tissue and replace them with dehydrating fluid.

- Solution is placed in increasing concentration of alcohol beginning with 50% to 100%. Each step takes about 2 to 3 hr. then two or three changes of absolute alcohol before proceeding to the clearing to the clearing stage.

## CLEARING:-

- This involves removing the alcohol and replacing it with a chemical that is miscible in both alcohol and paraffin. The chemical is xylene solution which will now infiltrate the tissue. Smaller tissues take up to an hour. Larger ones require 2 to 4 hr.

## EMBEDDING:-

- Paraffin infiltration, in this procedure tissue is dehydrated through a series of graded ethanol baths to displace the water. And then infiltrated with wax the infiltrated tissues are than embedded into wax block. The most commonly used waxes for infiltration are the commercial paraffin waxes.

## SECTIONING TISSUES:-

- Tissues are sectioned using a microtome. Turn on the water bath and temperature 35 to 37c. Use the deionized water. Place a fresh baled on the microtome. Blades may be used to section up to 10 blocks, but replace if sectioning becomes problematic. Insert the block into the microtome check so the wax block faces the blade and is aligned in the vertical plane.

- The blade should angled at 5`set the block b cutting it down to the desired tissue and discard the paraffin ribbon, if the block is ribbing well then cut another four section and pick them up with forceps or a fine paint brush and float them surface of the 37c temperature water bath.

- Float the section on to the surface of clean glass slide. If the block is not ribbon well then place it back in the ice block to cool off firm up the wax. If the specimen fragment when placed on the water bath then it may be too hot.

- Place the slide with paraffin section on the warming block in a 65 temperature oven for 20 min to bond the tissue to the glass. Slide can be stored or staining.

## STAINING:-

- Hematoxyline and Eosin (H&E) staining is the most common staining technique in histology. This use a combination two dyes, used for demonstration of nucleus and Cytoplasmic inclusions in clinical specimen.

## MOUNTING:-

- Stained sections are removed from xylene. Drain the excess xylene and mount on DPX or Canada balsom with a cover slip.

# URIN EXAMINATION

> ## Determination

Volume

## Normal finding

50ml to 200 ml

## Abnormal finding

> 500 ml

## Pathologic

Polyuria, Diabetes Mellitus

> ## Determination

Colour

## Normal finding

Pale yellow

## Pathologic

| | | |
|---|---|---|
| Dark yellow | - | Bilirubin |
| Brownish yellow | - | Post hepatic |
| White | - | Chyle, pus |
| Pink to red | - | hemoglobinuria, Febrile disease |
| Brownish Black | - | Alkaptonuria |
| Blue green | - | Presence biliverdin, Pseudomonas infection |

> ## Determination

Appearance

## Normal finding

Usually clear

## Pathologic

| | | |
|---|---|---|
| Turbid | - | No. of bacteria, WBC, Pus, epithelial cells. |
| Hazy | - | Mucus |
| Smoky | - | Red blood |
| Milky | - | Chyle |

## ➢ Determination

- Odor

## Normal finding

Aromatic

## Pathologic

Fruity Acidosis, Ketosis,  Diabetes mellitus

Ammoniacal          Cystitis

 Foul smelling          UTI, Coliform bacteria

## ➢ Determination

Reaction

## Normal finding

 Acidic PH   4.8-7.5

## Pathologic

| | | |
|---|---|---|
| PH less than 4.5 | - | Acidosis, Fevers, |
| more acidic urine | - | Ketosis |
| PH more than 7.5 | - | Severe vomiting, |
| Alkaline Urine | - | Obstructive gastric Ulcers. |

## ➢ Determination

Specific Gravity

## Normal finding

1.003 to 1.060

## Pathologic

Low sp gr.          -     Chronic nephritis , Diabetes insipidus

High sp.gr.         -     Diabetes mellitus ,Fever, Acute nephritis

> **Determination**

Proteins

## Normal finding

Absent

## Pathologic

Present     -     Heart disease, severe Diarrhoea

> **Determination**

Glucose

## Normal finding

Absent

## Pathologic

Present     -     Diabetes mellitus

> **Determination**

Urobilinogen

## Normal finding

Absent

## Pathologic

presents          Hepatic and post - Hepatic condition

> **Determination**

Bile salt And Bile pigment

## Normal finding

Absent

<u>**Pathologic**</u>

Present           -           Hepatic and post – Hepatic condition

➢ <u>**Determination**</u>

Blood

<u>**Normal finding**</u>

Absent

<u>**Pathologic**</u>

Present           -           Hematuria, renal Carcinoma, severe

Burns, hemolytic Transfusion.

➢ <u>**Determination**</u>

Ketone bodies

<u>**Normal finding**</u>

Absent

<u>**Pathologic**</u>

Present  -     Severe diabetes,  Fevers, Prolonged

Diarrhoea & Vomiting

➢ <u>**Determination**</u>

Nitrites

<u>**Normal finding**</u>

Negative

<u>**Pathologic**</u>

Positive     -      bacteriuria

➢ <u>**Determination**</u>

Pus

<u>**Normal finding**</u>

2to 3/HPF

## Pathologic

>5 cell/HPF   -      UTI, Pyuria, Stress

### ➢ Determination

Epithelial cells

### Normal finding

2 to 3/HPF

### Pathologic

>5cell/HPF   -      Tubular damage, Kidney transplant Rejection

### ➢ Determination

Cast

### Normal finding

Absent

### Pathologic

| | | |
|---|---|---|
| Present | - | Glomerular damage |
| Hyaline cast | - | Dehydration, exercise |
| Granular cast | - | Kidney disease |
| Fatty cast | - | Lipiduria |
| RBC cast | - | Bleeding into tubule |
| | | From the glomerulurus |
| WBC cast | - | Parenchymal infection |
| Tubular epithelial | - | Damage to the tubules Cast |

### ➢ Determination

Crystal  Acidic

### Normal finding

Absent

<u>**Pathologic**</u>

Present high level        -        Renal calculi.

> <u>**Determination**</u>

Parasites

<u>**Normal finding**</u>

Absent

<u>**Pathologic**</u>

Present                -        Trichomonas  Vaginalis

> **URINALYSIS**

- The three steps of urine formation

1) Filtration
2) Reabsorption
3) Secretion

**Filtration:-**

- The kidney is the body's blood filtering system. Blood vessels visit the kidney and enter capillaries called the glomerulus. The glomerulus is region of the kidney called the bowman's capsule. This is where filtration occurs.

- Blood is pushed through the tiny capillaries the high pressure forces some things to pass through the capillaries walls. The walls act as a sieve or filter.

**Re- absorption:-**

- The filtrate enters the kidney in the proximal tubule. This region of the kidney is special because many things can be removed from the filtrate. These valuable things are recollected or reabsorbed by the body.

**Secretion:-**

- The filtrate then passes through a really neat structure called the loop of Henle where it gains and loses water and salt. As it leaves the loop of Henle it enters the distal tubule, where secretion occurs.

**Collection of urine specimen** - Containers for the collection of urine should be wide mounted clean and dry.

**Amorphous urates:-**

- Yellow and granular precipitate

**Uric acid crystal:-**

- This crystal appear in several forms, multi coloured most commonly diamond shaped.

**Calcium oxalate:-**

- This crystal is most frequently observed in urine

**Crystal found in alkaline:-**

- Amorphous phosphates – fine granular precipitates

- Calcium carbonate – colourless spheres or dumbbell shaped

- Triple phosphate – crystals are colourless

**Crystal found in abnormal urine:-**

- Cystine – colour less, hexagonal

- Tyrosine – fine needle in clumps, yellow and silky

- Leucine – Yellow oily spheres

- Sulphonamide – Yellow brown

# STOOL EXAMINATION

**Introduction:-**

- A stool analysis is a test done on a faces sample to help diagnose certain condition affecting the digestive tract.

- These condition can include infection such as from parasite, viruses, and bacteria, Poor Nutrient absorption or cancer.

**Sample collect:-**

- A random stool sample can be taken.
- Collect the sample in clean, free container.
- Infants collect from the diaper.

**Precautions:-**

- Warm stool are better for the ova and parasite.
- Don`t refrigerator the stool for ova and parasites.
- Stool for ova and parasites can be collect in formalin and alcohol. these are used as a fixative.
- Semi- formed stool should be examined within 60 minutes of collection.
- Trophozoites degenerate in liquid stool rapidly so exam the stool 30 minutes.

**Indication:-**

- The presence of WBCs and RBCs.
- To find ova or parasites.
- To see the presence of fat for malabsorption syndrome.
- Colon cancer
- Ulceration of GI tract.
- Disease in the presence of diarrhoea and constipation.

**The stool is examined :-**

1) Grossly
2) Microscopically
3) Chemically

**1) Gross stool examination includes :-**

- Consistency
- Colour
- Quantity
- Odour
- Mucous

**2) Microscopic examination includes :-**

- Presence of leukocytes
- Presence of red blood cells
- Ova and parasites
- Presence of fat
- Presence of pus cells

**3) The chemical examination :-**

- Stool PH
- Reducing substance

**Consistency stool may be:-**

- Loosely formed stools
- Dry or hard stools
- Thin stool
- Diarrheal stool are watery
- Steatorrhea stool foul smells
- Constipated stool are firm and may be spherical and hard stool
- Ribbon like stool suggested the rectal narrowing or partial obstruction.

## Colour:-

- **Normal colour** - normal colour is due to the presence of stercobilinogen.

- **Yellow or green** – Green colour is seen in diarrhoea.

- **Black** - Black stool are due to bleeding of upper GI tract.

- **Maroon or pink** – this colour is from lower GI tract.

- **Clay coloured** – this stool are due to biliary obstruction.

- **Mucous** – mucous in the stool indicate constipation, colitis, or malignancy.

- **Pale colour with greasy** – appearance is due to pancreatic deficiency leading to malabsorption.

## Stool PH:-

- This depends upon the dietary intake.

- Normally stool is slightly acidic or alkaline depending on the diet.

## Alkaline stool seen in;-

- Colitis
- Diarrhoea
- Antibiotic therapy

## Acidic stool seen in;-

- Fat malabsorption
- Carbohydrate deficiency
- Disaccharide deficiency

## Microscopic examination:-

- Virus and parasites don't cause WBCs in the stool.

**Increased number of WBCs in the stool;**

- Bacillary dysentery
- Chronic ulcerative colitis
- Salmonella infection

**Absence of WBCs in the stool;**

- Cholera
- Viral diarrhoea
- Amoebic colitis
- Parasitic infection
- Toxigenic bacterial infection

**Presence of red blood cells in the stool can be;**

- cancer
- dysentery
- haemorrhoids

**Presence of fat;**

- malabsorption
- deficiency of pancreatic digestive enzyme
- Deficiency of bile.

# SEMEN EXAMINATION

- Semen analysis also known as a sperm count test, analysis the health and viability of man`s sperm.

- Sperm is the male gamete that is the male sex cell or the cell in males which has the capacity to fertilise an egg.

- Sperm are produced in the seminiferous tubes of the testes.

- the pituitary gland at the base of the brain causes testosterone to be produced in the testes. Testosterone cause sperm produced.

- The sperm production cycle takes approximately three months and a healthy man produces million of new sperm each day.

- Semen is the fluid containing sperm that`s released during ejaculation. Semen analysis measure three major factor of sperm health:-

- The number of sperm
- The shape of the sperm
- The movement of the sperm also known "sperm motility".

- Important to follow these instruction for accurate result.

- Avoid ejaculation for 24 to 72 hr before the test.
- Avoid alcohol, caffeine and drugs such as cocaine 2 to 5 days before the test.
- Avoid any hormone medication.

- Normal range: - 15 to 200 million / ml

**Sperm shape:-**

- A normal result for sperm shape is that more than 50% of sperm are normally shaped. If a man has greater than 50% of sperm that are abnormally shaped. This reduces his fertility.

**Movement:-**

- Normal result more than 50% of sperm must move normally an hour after ejaculation.

- Sperm movement or motility is important to fertility because sperm must travel to fertilize an egg.

**PH:-**

- A PH level should be between 7.2 and 7.8 to achieve a normal result.

- A PH level higher than 8.0 could indicate the donor has an infection.

- A result less than 7.0 could indicated the specimen is contaminated or that the man`s ejaculatory duct are blocked.

**Volume:-**

- The volume of semen for a normal result should be greater than 2 ml. A low semen volume could indicate a low amount of sperm to fertilize an egg.

**Sperm count:-**

- The sperm count in a normal semen analysis should be between 20 million to over 200 million. This result is also known as sperm density. If this number is low conceiving can be more difficult.

**Appearance:-**

- The appearance should be whitish to gray and opalescent. Semen that has a red brown tint could indicate the presence of blood while a yellow tint cloud indicate jaundice.

**Abnormal results cloud indicates the following:-**

- Infertility
- Infection
- Hormonal imbalance
- Disease such as diabetes

- Gene effect
- Exposure to radiation

**Liquefaction time :-**

- Immediately after ejaculation seminal fluid is thick mucus like substance in which sperm are suspended. Normal seminal fluid will change to watery liquid within 15 to 60 minutes of ejaculation.

**Normozoospermia:-**

- Normozoospermia is the presence of normal sperm in semen upon semen analysis.

**Oligozoospermia :-**

- Oligozoospermia refer to semen with a low concentration of sperm and is common finding In male infertility.

**Asthenozoospermia:-**

- This condition is characterized by reduced motility or absent sperm motility in the fresh ejaculate.

**Teratozoospermia:-**

- Teratospermia is a semen alteration in which there are a large number of spermatozoa With abnormal morphology. It is a sperm condition that may lead to serious Consequence Such as male infertility.

**Azoospermia:-**

- Azoospermia is the complete absence of any sperm in man semen. Azoospermia is a major cause of male infertility.

**Aspermia:-**

- The absence of spermatozoa in the semen or the inability to ejaculate semen.

Obstructive Aspermia is due to the blockage of the vas deferens on both sides.

**Necrozoospermia:-**

- When all the sperm are dead in fresh semen sample. Incomplete Necrozoospermia is when many but not all of the sperm in semen sample are dead. Typically when less than 45% but more than 5% are viable.

# SPUTUM EXAMINATION

**Sputum examination**

- Sputum it contains approximately 95% water and 5% total solid. The solids are primarily carbohydrates, proteins, lipids, DNA.

**Specimen collection:-**

- Early morning specimen collect.

- Sterile container wide mouth with screw cap.

- The sputum must be coughed up from the lungs or bronchi and placed carefully in the container.

> **TEST**

Quantity

**NORMAL**

2-5 ml

**ABNORMAL**

24hr over 100ml  OR  500 ml

**CLINICAL SIGNIFICANCE**

Bronchiectasis, lung abscess,  Amoebic abscess

> **TEST**

Colour

**NORMAL**

Colourless, clear

**ABNORMAL**

Different colour

| | | |
|---|---|---|
| Yellow | - | Pus & Epithelial cells |
| Greenish | - | Pseudomonas infection |
| Black | - | Coal dust |
| Bright red | - | recent haemorrhage, Pulmonary infection, Pulmonary tuberculosis |

> **TEST**

Consistency

**NORMAL**

watery & Opalescent

**ABNORMAL**

Different Consistency

**CLINICAL SIGNIFICANCE**

| | | |
|---|---|---|
| Mucoid | - | Whooping cough, asthma |
| Bloody | - | Tuberculosis, carcinoma lungs |
| Mucopurolent | - | Mucus & pus found in lungs |

# ROUTINE EXAMINATION OF FLUID

- Four types of fluids

1) Pleural fluid (Around lungs fluid).
2) Pericardial fluid (Around heart cavity fluid).
3) Peritoneal fluid (Ascitic) (Around abdomen pelvic fluid).
4) Synovial fluid (Around Joints fluid).

| **FLUID** | **COLOUR** | **APPEARANCE** | **CLINICAL CONDITION** |
|---|---|---|---|
| Pleural | Pale & | Clear | Normal |
| Fluid | Straw colour | | |
| | | Turbidity | Increase in cells & Debris |
| | | Cloudy | It indicates inflammation, Viral or bacterial infection |
| | | Bloody | Traumatic tap, pancreatitis, Tuberculosis, heart failure. |
| | | Milky | Pseudochylous effusion, Rheumatoid arthritis. |
| Pericardial Fluid | Straw colour | Clear | Normal |
| | | Cloudy | Myxedema, post myocardial Infraction, septic condition. |

| | | Bloody | Tuberculosis, aortic syndrome |
|---|---|---|---|
| Pericardial Fluid | Straw colour | Clear | Normal |
| | | Turbid | Appendicitis, pancreatitis |
| | | Pale yellow | Hepatic vein obstruction Cirrhosis, congestive heart Failure. |
| | | Greenish | Cholecystitis, perforated Gall Bladder. |
| | | Milky | Parasitic infection, Carcinoma, Lyphoma |
| | | Blood | Ruptured spleen, Ruptured liver. |
| Synovial Fluid | Yellow & Viscous | Clear | Normal |
| | | Turbid | Septic arthritis. |
| | | Bloody | Traumatic tap. |

9 789388 393126